HUMAN CROSS-SECTIONAL ANATOMY
Atlas of Body Sections and CT Images

Harold Ellis CBE MA DM MCh FRCS FRCOG
Clinical Anatomist, Department of Anatomy
University of Cambridge
Downing Street, Cambridge CB2 3DY

Bari M Logan MA FMA Hon MBIE
Prosector, Department of Anatomy
University of Cambridge
Downing Street, Cambridge CB2 3DY

Adrian Dixon MA MD MRCP FRCR DMRD
Lecturer
Department of Radiology
University of Cambridge;

Honorary Consultant Radiologist
Addenbrooke's Hospital
Hills Road, Cambridge CB2 2QQ

and

Fellow/Director of Studies in Medicine,
Peterhouse, Cambridge

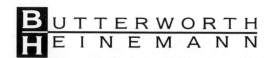
BUTTERWORTH
HEINEMANN

Butterworth-Heinemann Ltd
Linacre House, Jordan Hill, Oxford OX2 8DP

$\mathcal{R}$ A member of the Reed Elsevier group

OXFORD   LONDON   BOSTON   MUNICH   NEW DELHI   SINGAPORE
SYDNEY   TOKYO   TORONTO   WELLINGTON

First published 1991
Reprinted 1993

© Butterworth-Heinemann Ltd 1991

British Library Cataloguing in Publication Data
Ellis, Harold
    Human cross-sectional anatomy: Atlas of body
    sections and CT images.
    I. Title   II. Logan, Bari   III. Dixon, Adrian
    611.0022

ISBN 0 7506 1241 X

Library of Congress Cataloging in Publication Data
A CIP record for this book is available from the Library of Congress

Composition by Genesis Typesetting, Laser Quay, Rochester, Kent
Printed in Scotland by Cambus Litho Ltd, Glasgow
Bound in Scotland by Hunter and Foulis Ltd, Edinburgh

Preface

The study of sectional anatomy of the human body goes back to the earliest days of systematic topographical anatomy. The beautiful drawings of the sagittal sections of the male and female trunk and of the pregnant uterus by Leonardo da Vinci (1452–1519) are well known. Among his figures (which were based on some 30 dissections) are a number of transverse sections of the lower limb. These constitute the first known examples of the use of cross-sections for the study of gross anatomy and anticipate modern technique by several hundred years. In the absence of hardening reagents or methods of freezing it was only seldom used by Leonardo (O'Malley and Saunders, 1952). Andreas Vesalius pictured transverse sections of the brain in his *Fabrica* published in 1543; and in the 17th century portrayals of sections of various parts of the body, including the brain, eye and the genitalia were made by Vidius, Bartholin, de Graaf and others. Drawings of sagittal section anatomy were used to illustrate surgical works in the 18th century – for example, those of Antonio Scarpa of Pavia and Peter Camper of Leyden. William Smellie, one of the fathers of British midwifery, published his magnificent *Anatomical Tables* in 1754, mostly drawn by Riemsdyk, which mainly comprised sagittal sections. William Hunter's illustrations of the human gravid uterus are also well known.

The main obstacle to detailed sectional anatomical studies was, of course, the problem of fixation of tissues during the cutting process. De Riemer, a Dutch anatomist, published an atlas of human transverse sections in 1818 which were obtained by freezing the cadaver. The other technique which was developed during the early 19th century was the use of gypsum to envelop the parts and to retain the organs in their anatomical position – a method used by the Weber brothers in 1836.

Pirogoff, the well-known Russian surgeon, produced his massive five volume cross-sectional anatomy between 1852 and 1859, which was illustrated with 213 plates. He used the freezing technique, which he claimed (falsely, as noted above) to have introduced as a novel method of fixation.

The second half of the 19th century saw the publication of a number of excellent sectional atlases, and photographic reproductions were used by Braun as early as 1875. Perhaps the best known atlas of this era in the UK was that of Sir William Macewen, Professor of Surgery in Glasgow, and published in 1893. Entitled *Atlas of Head Sections*, it comprised a series of coronal, sagittal and transverse sections of the head in adult and child. This was the first atlas to show the skull and brain together in detail. Macewen intended his atlas to be of practical, clinical value and wrote in his preface 'the surgeon who is about to perform an operation on the brain has in these cephalic sections a means of refreshing his memory regarding the position of the various structures he is about to encounter'. This from the surgeon who first proved, in his treatment of cerebral abscess, that clinical neurological localization could be correlated with accurate surgical exposure.

The use of formalin as a hardening and preserving fluid was introduced by Gerota in 1895, and it was soon found that thorough perfusion of the vascular system of the cadaver enabled satisfactory sections to be obtained of the formalin-hardened material. The early years of the 20th century saw the publication of a number of atlases based on this technique. Perhaps the most comprehensive and beautifully executed of these was *A Cross-section Anatomy* produced by Eycleshymer and Schoemaker of St Louis University. This was first published in 1911, and its masterly historical introduction in the 1930 edition provides an extensive bibliography of sectional anatomy.

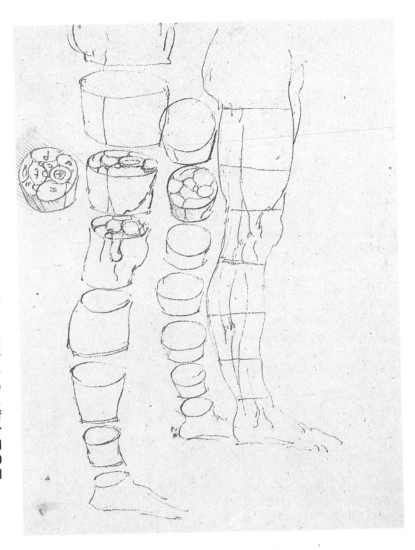

Leonardo da Vinci – The right leg of a man measured, then cut into sections
Source: Windsor Castle Royal Library © 1991 Her Majesty The Queen

The importance of cross-sectional anatomy

Successive authors of atlases on cross-sectional anatomy have emphasized the value to the anatomist and to the surgeon of being able to view the body in this dimension. It is always difficult to consider three dimensions in the mind's eye; to be able to view the relationships of the viscera and fascial planes in transverse section helps to clarify the conventional appearances of the body's structure as seen in the operating theatre, in the dissecting room and in the textbook.

The introduction of modern scanning techniques, especially ultrasound and (even more) computed tomography, has enormously expanded the already considerable importance of cross-sectional anatomy. The radiologist, neurologist, internist, chest physician and oncologist, as well as specialists in the various fields of surgery, have had to re-educate themselves in the appearances and relationships of anatomical structures in transverse section. Indeed, precise diagnosis, as well as the detailed planning of therapy (for example, the ablative surgery of extensive cancer) and of interventional radiology, often depends on the cross-sectional anatomical approach.

This atlas combines two presentations of cross-sectional anatomy, that of the dissecting room and that of computed tomography. The two series are matched to each other as closely as possible on opposite pages. Students of anatomy, surgeons, clinicians and radiologists should find the illustrations of anatomical cross-sections (obtained by the most modern techniques of preparation and photographic reproduction) and the equivalent cuts on computed tomography (obtained on state-of-the-art apparatus) both interesting and rewarding.

Preservation of cadavers

Preservation of the cadavers used for the sections in this atlas was by standard embalming technique, using two electric motor pumps set at a maximum pressure rate of 15 p.s.i. Preservative fluid was circulated through the arterial system via two cannulae inserted into the femoral artery of one leg. A partial flushing of blood was effected from the accompanying femoral vein by the insertion of a large bore drainage tube.

After the successful acceptance of 20 litres of preservative fluid, local injection by automatic syringe was carried out on those areas which remained unaffected. On average, approximately 30 litres of preservative fluid was used to preserve each cadaver.

Following preservation, the cadavers were stored in thick-gauge polythene tubes and refrigerated to a temperature of 51°F (10.6°C), for a minimum 16-week period before sectioning. This period allowed the preservative solution to saturate thoroughly the body tissues, resulting in a highly satisfactory state of preservation.

The chemical formula for the preservative solution (Logan et al., 1989) is:

Methylated spirit 64 op	12.5	litres
Phenol liquified 80%	2.5	litres
Formaldehyde solution 38%	1.5	litres
Glycerine BP	3.5	litres

The resultant working strength of each constituent is:

Methylated spirit	55%
Glycerine	12%
Phenol	10%
Formaldehyde solution	3%

The advantages of this particular preservative solution are that (1) a state of soft preservation is achieved; (2) the low formaldehyde solution content obviates excessive noxious fumes during dissection; (3) a degree of natural tissue colour is maintained which benefits photography; and (4) mould growth does not occur on either whole cadavers thus preserved, or their subsequent prosected and stored parts.

Sectioning

Four preserved cadavers, two male and two female, were used to produce the 90 cross-sections illustrated in this atlas.

The parts to be sectioned were deep-frozen to a temperature of −40°C for a minimum three-day period immediately prior to sectioning.

Sectioning was carried out on a purpose-built AEW 600 stainless steel bandsaw (AEW Engineering Co. Ltd, Horizon Works, Dereham Road, Costessey, Norwich, NR5 0SA, England). The machine is equipped with a 10 h.p., three-phase electric motor which is capable of producing a constant blade speed of 6000 feet per minute. A fine-toothed (four skip) stainless steel blade was used, 19 mm in depth and precisely 1 mm in thickness (including tooth set). The design and precision manufacture of the machine results, during operation, in the loss of only 1 mm of material between each section.

Sections were taken from the cadavers to the following thickness of cut:

Head	1 cm serial
Neck	1.5 cm serial
Thorax	2 cm serial
Abdomen	2 cm serial
Pelvis male	2 cm serial
Pelvis female	2 cm serial
Lower limb	at selected levels
Upper limb	at selected levels

Computed tomography (CT)

Ever since the invention of CT by Hounsfield (1973) there has been renewed interest in sectional anatomy. Despite the high cost, CT systems are now widely used throughout the more affluent countries. Radiologists in particular have had to go through a rapid learning process. Several excellent sectional CT-anatomy books have been produced. However, more modern CT technology allows a wider range of structures to be demonstrated with better image quality, mainly due to improved spatial resolution and shorter data acquisition times. Hence the justification for yet another atlas which correlates anatomical and CT images.

The images in this volume have been obtained on a Siemens Somatom Plus which was installed in Addenbrooke's Hospital, Cambridge in November 1989. The imaging protocols used in our unit have long been established (Dixon, 1983a); these have not substantially changed with the advent of the new machine. Oral contrast medium is routinely given for abdominopelvic studies; thus the stomach and small bowel usually appear opaque. Contrast medium is often administered per rectum before a pelvic study. The use of intravenous contrast medium can also provide additional information, and thus in some sections the vessels appear opaque.

Precise correlation between the cadaveric sections and the clinical images is very difficult to obtain in practice, as no two patients are quite the same shape! The distribution of fat, particularly in the abdomen, varies from patient to patient and between the sexes (Dixon, 1983b). Furthermore, there are the inevitable physiological discrepancies between cadaveric slices and images obtained in vivo. These are especially noticeable in the juxta-diaphragmatic region. In particular, the vertebral levels do not quite correlate because of the effect of inspiration; all intrathoracic structures are better displayed on images obtained at suspended inspiration. Furthermore, in order to obtain as precise a correlation as possible, some CT images are not quite of optimal quality.

A further difficulty which is encountered when attempting to correlate the two sets of images is caused by the fact that CT involves ionizing radiation. The radiation dose has to be kept to the minimum which answers the clinical problem: thus it is not always easy to find photogenic examples of normal anatomy for all parts of the body. This is especially true in the limbs, which are relatively infrequently studied by CT.

Some knowledge of the X-ray attenuation of normal structures is useful to assist interpretation of the images. The Hounsfield scale extends from air, which measures −1000 HU (Hounsfield Units), through pure water at 0 HU to beyond +1000 HU for dense cortical bone. Most soft tissues are in the range +35 to +70 HU (kidney, muscle, liver, etc). Fat provides useful negative contrast at around −100 HU. The displayed image can appear very different depending on the chosen window width (the spread of the grey scale) and the window level (the centre of the grey scale). These differences are especially apparent in Section 8 (the thorax) where the images are displayed both at soft tissue settings (window 400, level +20 HU) and at lung settings (window approx. 1250, level −850 HU). Such image manipulation merely requires alteration of the stored electronic data at the viewing console, where any parameters can be chosen. The 'hard copy' photographic record of the electronic data is always a rather poor representation. Indeed, in clinical practice, it may be difficult to display all structures and some lesions on hard copy film.

Orientation of sections and images

A concerted effort over the last few years, mainly led by American radiologists, has meant that axial cross-sectional images are now viewed in a standard, conventional manner. Hitherto there was wide variation which led to considerable confusion and even medico-legal complications.

ALL cross-sectional images in clinical practice are now viewed as shown in Figure A; that is from 'below' and 'looking up'. This is

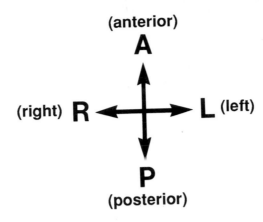

Figure B

the logical method, insofar that the standard way in which a doctor approaches the examination of the supine patient is from the right hand, foot end of a couch. The image is thus in the correct orientation for the doctor's palpating right hand. For example, he or she has to 'reach across' the image to find the spleen, exactly as would happen during the clinical examination of the abdomen. Similarly, for the head, the right eye is the one more accessible for right-handed ophthalmoscopy. Thus, all axial sections should be considered, learned and even displayed with an orientation logo shown in Figure B. This is the same orientation as that used for other images (e.g. a chest radiograph). Here again, the right of the patient is on the viewer's left, just as if the clinician was about to shake hands with the patient.

Happily there is now world-wide agreement over this matter with regard to clinical imaging. Furthermore, many anatomy books have adopted this approach so that students learn this method from outset. Ideally, embryologists and members of all other disciplines concerned with anatomical orientation should ultimately conform to this method.

The orientation logo in Figure B is suitable for the head, neck, thorax, abdomen and pelvis. However in the limbs, when only one limb is displayed, further clarification is required. All depends on whether a right or left limb is being examined. To assist this quandary, a medial (M) and a lateral (L) marker is provided and is shown in Figure C. In this volume a left limb has been used throughout. Again, viewing is as from 'below'.

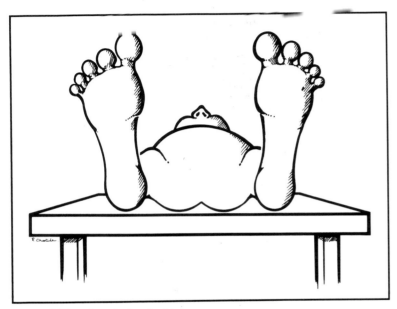

Figure A View from below looking up

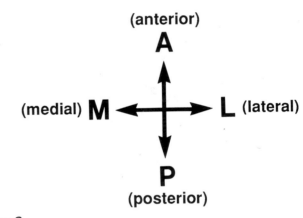

Figure C

Notes on the Atlas

This atlas presents in sequence transverse sections of the cadaver with corresponding CT images. The logical sequence should enable the student to find the desired anatomical level with ease.

The numbers placed on the colour photographs and on the line drawings which accompany each CT image match and the key to these numbers is given on the accompanying list on each page spread. Where numbers appear below the line on the key, these refer to features which are apparent only on the CT image.

Brief notes accompany each section and refer to important anatomical and CT features.

In the majority of sections, bilateral structures have been labelled only on one side. This has been done in order to allow readers to have an unobscured view of structures and to put their own anatomical knowledge to the test.

A series of views of a minimally dissected brain is provided in order to clarify the orientation of cerebral topography in the series of head sections.

The colour photographs of the brain dissections and of the sections of the upper and lower limb are of natural size. Those of the head and neck sections have been slightly reduced and still

greater reduction has been used in the thorax, abdomen and pelvis series in order to fit the page format. All the CT images are of the size seen on the films used in current clinical practice.

An extra double-page spread of CT images of the mediastinum has been included in order to show the features of this important anatomical area in more detail than is demonstrated in the standard CT.

At the end of the abdomen series, which was prepared from a male subject, two female sections have been added for comparison.

References

Dixon, A. K. (1983a) *Body CT: a handbook*. Churchill Livingstone, Edinburgh

Dixon, A. K. (1983b) Abdominal fat assessed by computed tomography: sex difference in distribution. *Clinical Radiology*, **34**, 189–191

Eycleshymer, A. C. and Schoemaker, D. M. (1930) *A Cross-Section Anatomy*. Appleton, New York

Hounsfield, G. N. (1973) Computerized transverse axial scanning (tomography). *British Journal of Radiology*, **46**, 1016–1022

Logan, B. M., Watson, M. and Tattersall, R. (1989) A basic synopsis of the 'Cambridge' procedure for the preservation of whole human cadavers. *Institute of Anatomical Sciences Journal*, No 3, 25

Logan, B. M., Liles, R. P. and Bolton, I. (1990) A photographic technique for teaching topographical anatomy from whole body transverse sections. *The Journal of Audio Visual Media in Medicine*, **13** (No 2), 45–48

O'Malley, C. D. and Saunders, J. B. (1952) *Leonardo da Vinci on the human body*. Schuman, New York

Acknowledgements

Dissecting room staff

For skilled technical assistance in the preservation and sectioning of the cadavers

Mr M. Watson, Senior Technician
Mr R. Tattersall, Technician
Mr M. O'Hannan, Porter
} Anatomy Department, University of Cambridge

Audio visual unit

For photographic expertise

Mr J. Bashford
Mr R. Liles, LMPA
Mr I. Bolton
Mr A. Newman
} Anatomy Department, University of Cambridge

For excellent art work and graphics

Mrs R. Chesterton

Secretarial

For typing of manuscript

Miss J. McLachlan and Miss A. J. J. Burton, Anatomy Department, University of Cambridge

Printing of colour photographs

Simon Irwin of Streamline Colour Labs, Cambridge

Annotation of central nervous system (brain and head sections)

Dr Roger Lemon, Lecturer, Anatomy Department, University of Cambridge

Computed tomography

For performing many of the CT images

Mrs B. Housden, DCR
Mrs L. Clements, DCR
Radiographers, Addenbrooke's Hospital, Cambridge
Many radiological colleagues provided useful advice

The authors would also like to thank the staff at Butterworth–Heinemann for their help and advice in the production of this book.

MALE

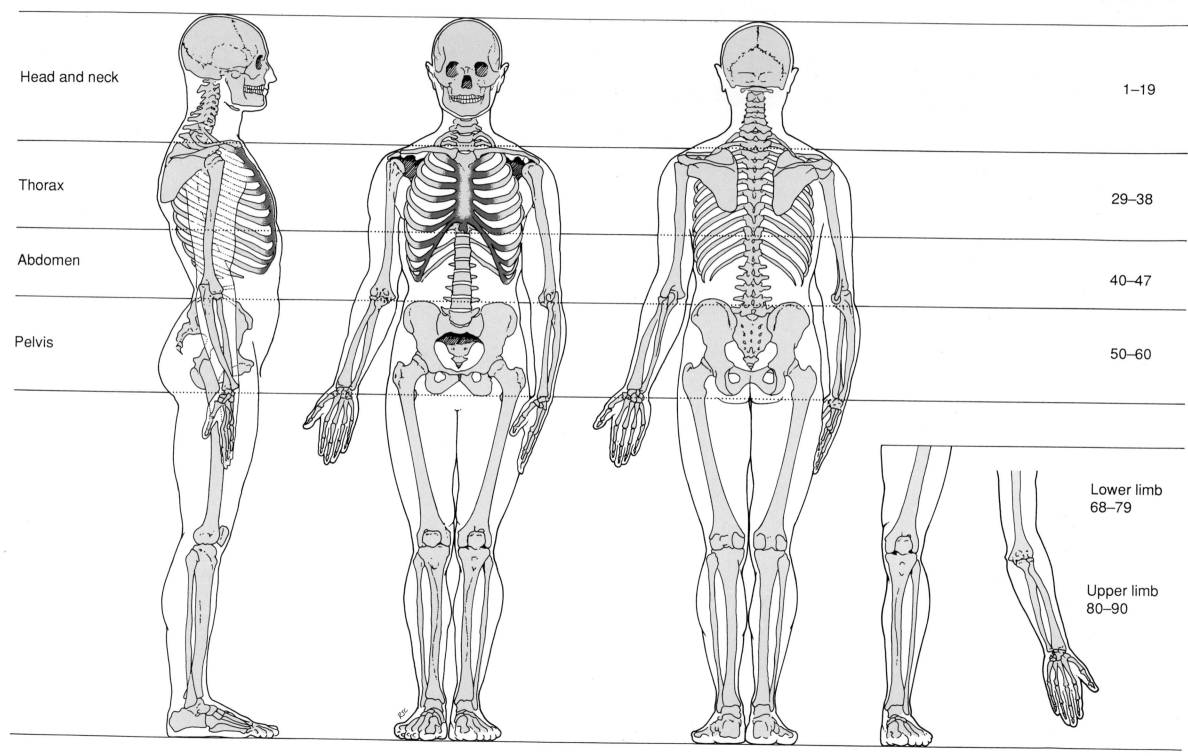

Head and neck — 1–19

Thorax — 29–38

Abdomen — 40–47

Pelvis — 50–60

Lower limb 68–79

Upper limb 80–90

FEMALE

	Sections
Head and neck	20–28
Thorax	39
Abdomen	48–49
Pelvis	61–67

HEAD SECTIONS

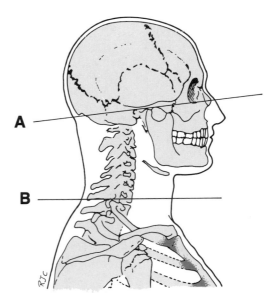

A   The radiographic base line used for cranial sections and images in this atlas has been selected as that running from the inferior orbital margin to the external auditory meatus. This allows most of the brain to be demonstrated without excessive bony artefact.

B   For sections and images of the neck and the rest of the body a true axial plane has been used.

The Brain

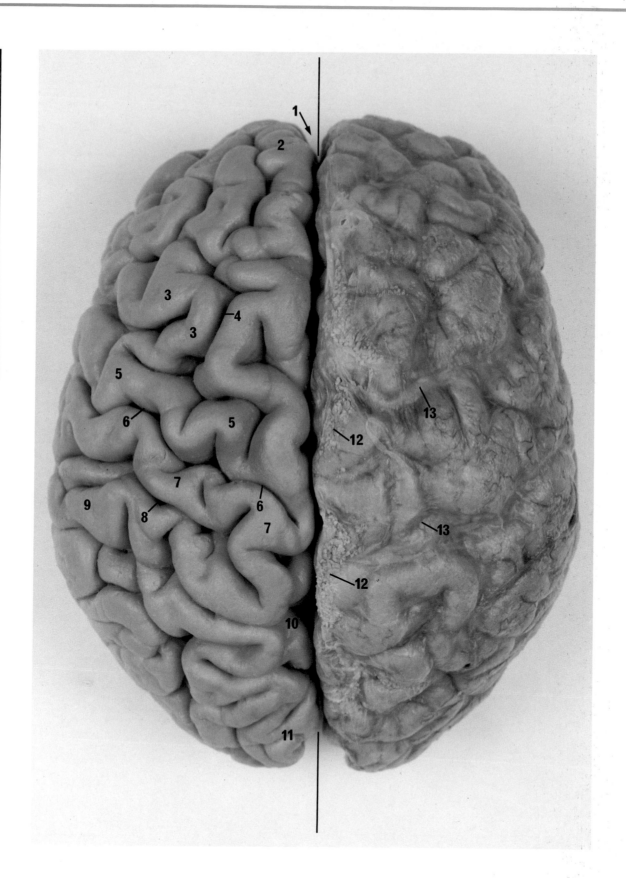

C Right cerebral hemisphere, cerebellum and brain stem. From below with the arachnoid mater and blood vessels intact

1 Longitudinal cerebral fissure (arrowed)
2 Frontal pole
3 Inferior surface of frontal pole
4 Temporal pole
5 Inferior surface of temporal pole
6 Internal carotid artery
7 Optic chiasma
8 Infundibulum
9 Parahippocampal gyrus
10 Basilar artery
11 Labyrinthine artery
12 Right vertebral artery
13 Medulla oblongata
14 Tonsil of cerebellum
15 Cerebellar hemisphere
16 Occipital pole

D Left cerebral hemisphere, cerebellum and brain stem. From below with the arachnoid mater and blood vessels removed

17 Orbital gyri
18 Olfactory bulb
19 Olfactory tract (I)
20 Medial olfactory stria
21 Lateral olfactory stria
22 Inferior temporal sulcus
23 Optic nerve (II)
24 Collateral sulcus
25 Optic tract
26 Oculomotor nerve (III)
27 Mamillary body
28 Pons
29 Trochlear nerve (IV)
30 Trigeminal nerve (V)
31 Abducent nerve (VI)
32 Facial nerve (VII)
33 Vestibulocochlear nerve (VIII)
34 Flocculus
35 Glossopharyngeal nerve (IX)
36 Vagus nerve (X)
37 Hypoglossal nerve (XII)
38 Accessory nerve (XI)

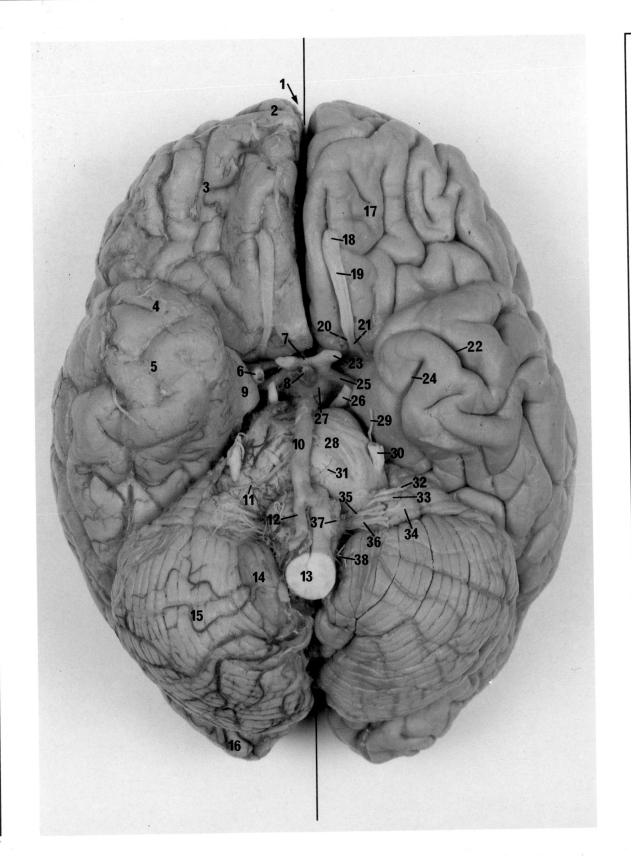

The Brain

E From the left with the arachnoid mater and blood vessels
intact

1 Rolandic artery (in central sulcus)
2 Superior anastomotic vein (Troland)
3 Superior cerebral veins
4 Lateral fissure
5 Inferior anastomotic vein (Labbé)
6 Superior cerebellar artery
7 Basilar artery
8 Vertebral artery

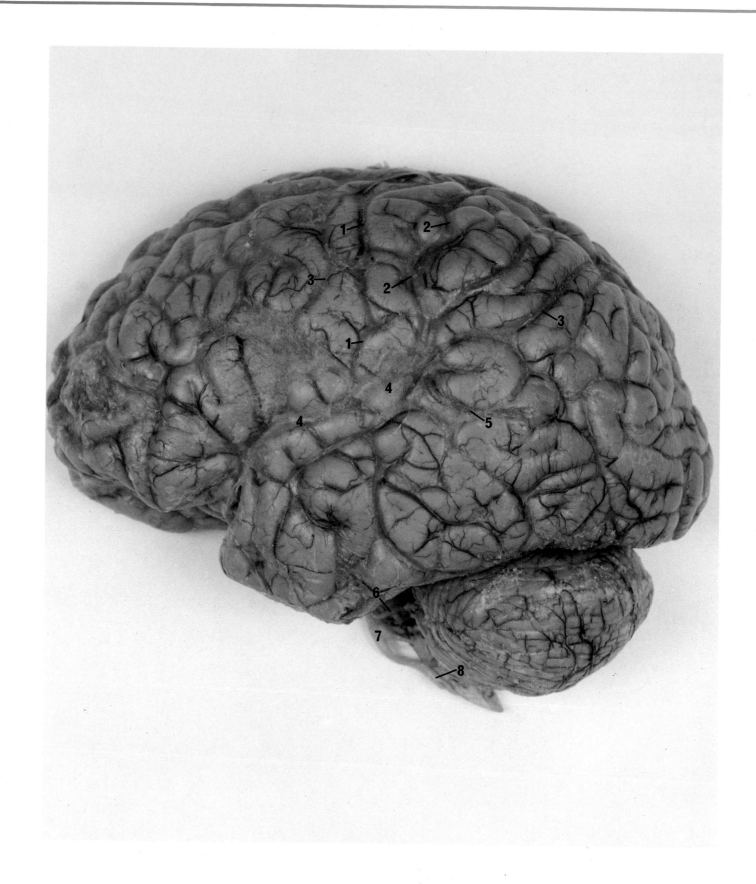

12

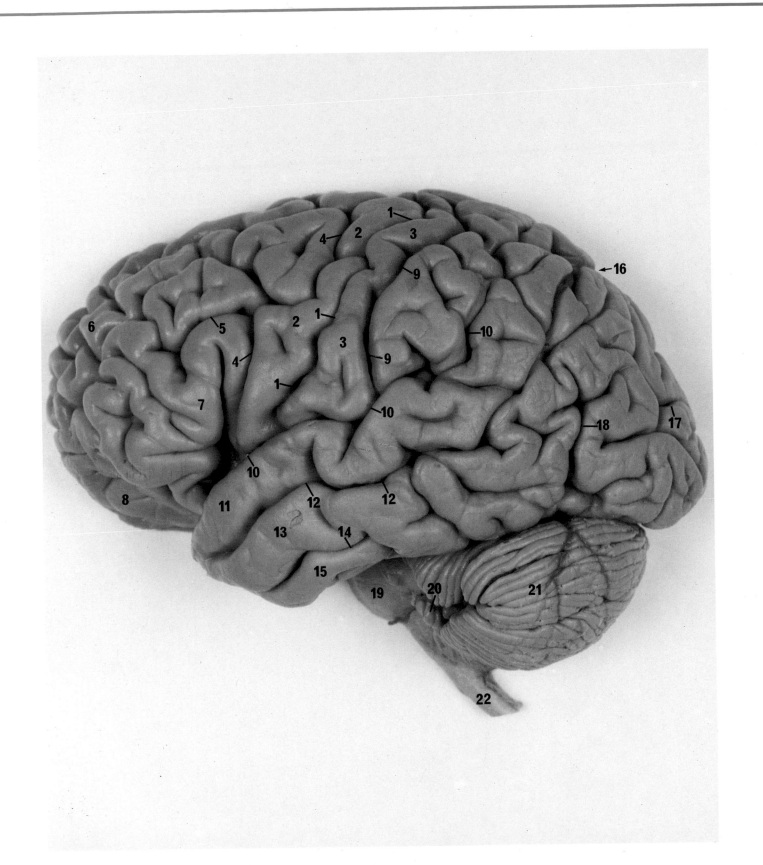

**F From the left with the arach-
noid mater and blood vessels
removed**

1 Central sulcus
2 Precentral gyrus
3 Postcentral gyrus
4 Precentral sulcus
5 Inferior frontal sulcus
6 Superior frontal gyrus
7 Inferior frontal gyrus
8 Orbital gyri
9 Postcentral sulcus
10 Lateral fissure
11 Superior temporal gyrus
12 Superior temporal sulcus
13 Middle temporal gyrus
14 Inferior temporal sulcus
15 Inferior temporal gyrus
16 Parieto-occipital fissure (arrowed)
17 Lunate sulcus
18 Anterior occipital sulcus
19 Pons
20 Flocculus
21 Cerebellar hemisphere
22 Medulla oblongata

The Brain

G A median sagittal section. The left half, from the right, with the arachnoid mater and blood vessels intact

1 Callosomarginal artery
2 Pericallosal artery
3 Calcarine artery
4 Posterior cerebral artery
5 Anterior cerebral artery
6 Orbital artery
7 Basilar artery
8 Anterior inferior cerebellar artery
9 Left vertebral artery

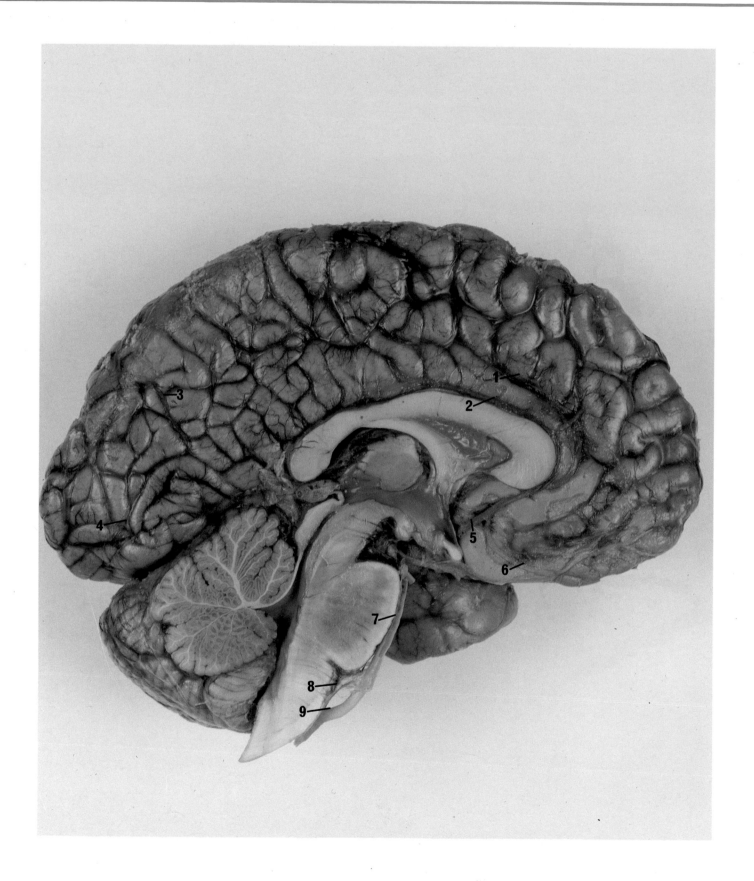

H A median sagittal section. The left half, from the right, with the arachnoid mater and blood vessels removed

1 Superior frontal gyrus
2 Cingulate sulcus
3 Cingulate gyrus
4 Callosal sulcus
5 Corpus callosum – body
6 Corpus callosum – genu
7 Corpus callosum – splenium
8 Fornix
9 Caudate nucleus (head) in wall of lateral ventricle
10 Choroid plexus, third ventricle
11 Interventricular foramen (Monro)
12 Thalamus
13 Massa intermedia
14 Anterior commissure
15 Pineal body
16 Posterior commissure
17 Superior colliculus
18 Aqueduct (of Sylvius)
19 Inferior colliculus
20 Mesencephalon
21 Hypothalamus
22 Mamillary body
23 Infundibulum
24 Uncus
25 Optic nerve (II)
26 Oculomotor nerve (III)
27 Trochlear nerve (IV)
28 Parahippocampal gyrus
29 Rhinal sulcus
30 Pons
31 Pontine tegmentum
32 Fourth ventricle
33 Nodulus
34 Anterior lobe of cerebellum
35 Parieto-occipital fissure
36 Calcarine sulcus
37 Cerebellar hemisphere
38 Tonsil of cerebellum
39 Inferior cerebellar peduncle
40 Pyramid
41 Medulla oblongata

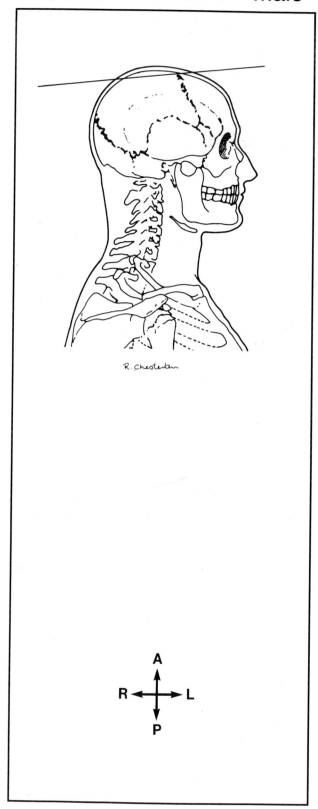

R. Chesterton

A
R ← → L
P

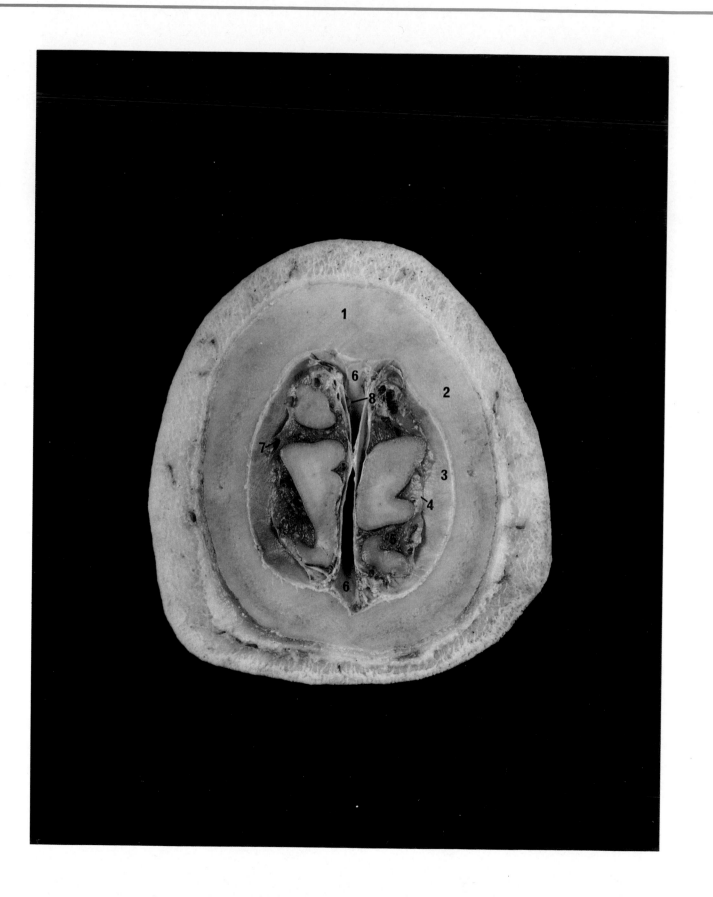

1 Frontal bone
2 Parietal bone
3 Dura mater
4 Arachnoid mater
5 Pia mater
6 Superior sagittal sinus
7 Superior cerebral vein
8 Arachnoid granulation

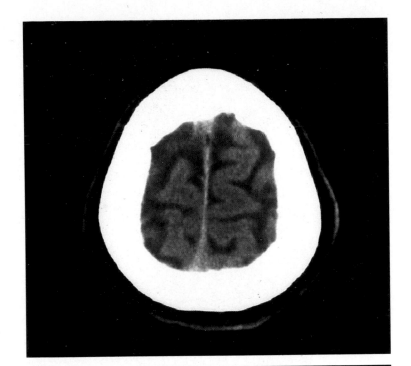

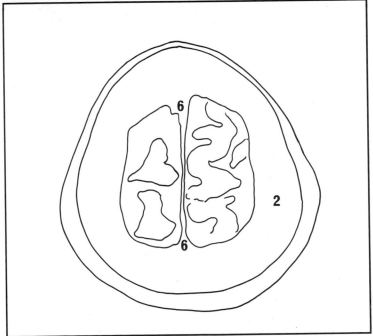

NOTES

This section passes through the apex of the skull vault and traverses the parietal bones (2) and the superior portion of the frontal bone (1).

The dura mater which lines the inner aspect of the skull comprises an outer, or endosteal, layer or endocranium (3) (which is, in fact, the periosteum which lines the inner aspect of the skull) and an inner, or meningeal, layer (4). Most of the intracranial venous sinuses are formed as clefts between these two layers, as demonstrated in this section by the superior sagittal sinus (6). The exceptions to this rule are the inferior sagittal sinus and the straight sinus, which are clefts within the meningeal layer.

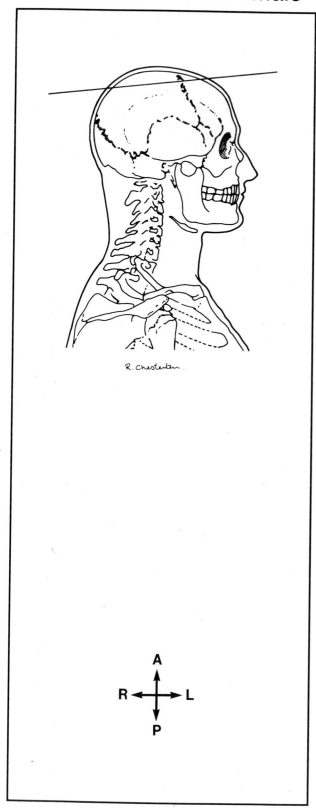

R. Chesterton

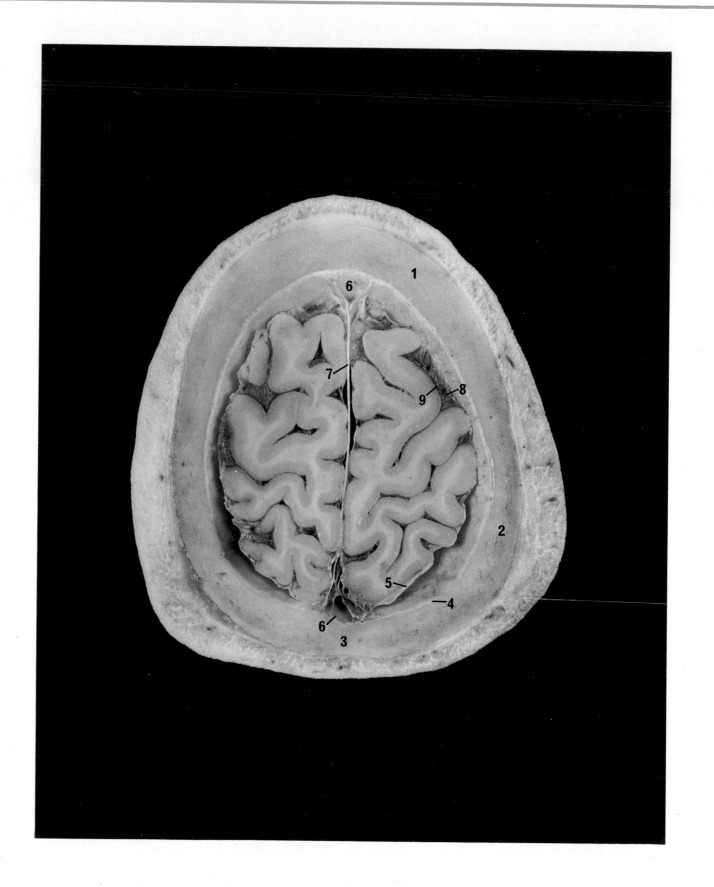

1 Frontal bone
2 Parietal bone
3 Sagittal suture
4 Dura mater
5 Arachnoid mater
6 Superior sagittal sinus
7 Falx cerebri
8 Subarachnoid space
9 Pia mater

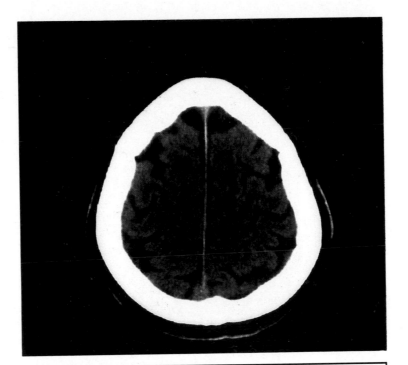

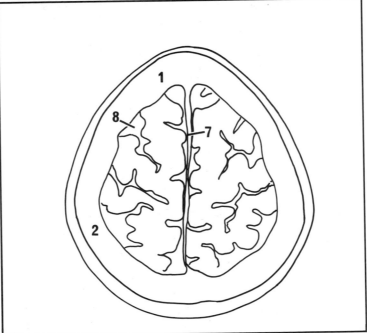

NOTES

This section, at a deeper plane through the skull vault, demonstrates the falx cerebri (7), which is formed as a double fold of the inner, meningeal, layer of the dura mater (5) and which forms the dural septum between the cerebral hemispheres.

The inner layer of the dura is lined by the delicate arachnoid mater. The pia mater (9) is vascular and invests the brain, spinal cord, cranial nerves and the spinal nerve roots. It remains in close contact with the surface of the brain, including the depths of the cerebral sulci and fissures.

Over the convexities of the brain, the pia and arachnoid are in close contact. Over the cerebral sulci and the cisterns of the brain base, the pia and arachnoid are separated by the subarachnoid space (8), which contains cerebrospinal fluid. This space is traversed by a fine spider's web of fibres (*arachnoid*: pertaining to the spider).

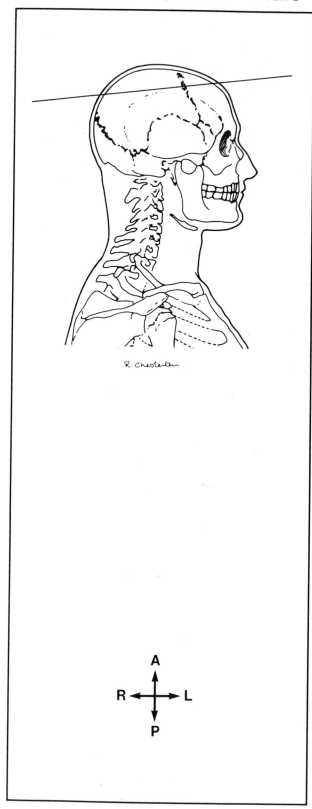

R. Chesterton

A
R ← → L
P

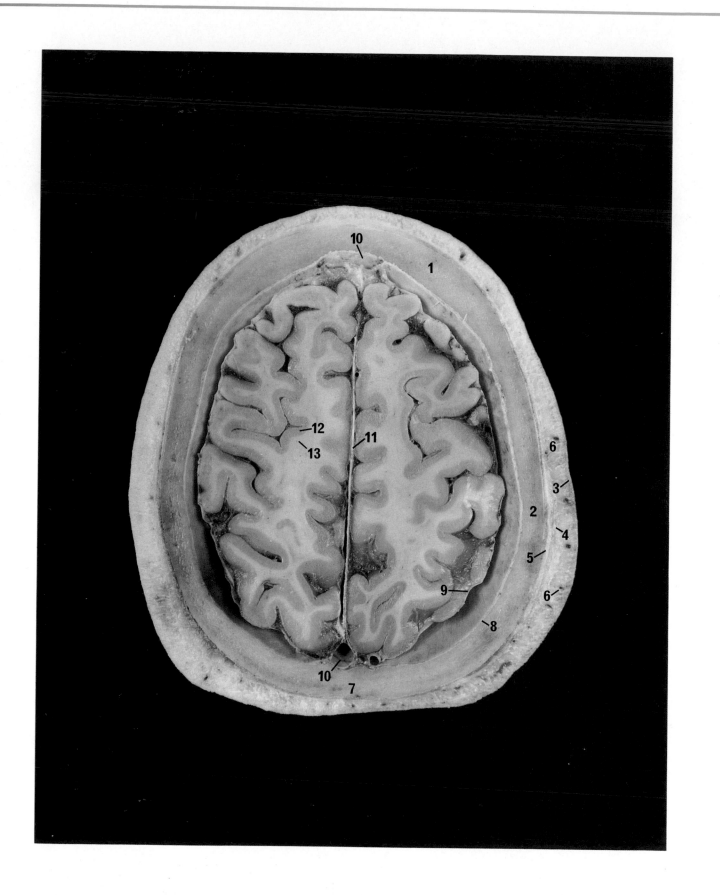

1 Frontal bone
2 Parietal bone
3 Skin and dense subcutaneous tissue
4 Epicranial aponeurosis (galea aponeurotica)
5 Pericranium
6 Branches of superficial temporal artery
7 Sagittal suture
8 Dura mater
9 Arachnoid mater
10 Superior sagittal sinus
11 Falx cerebri
12 Grey matter
13 White matter

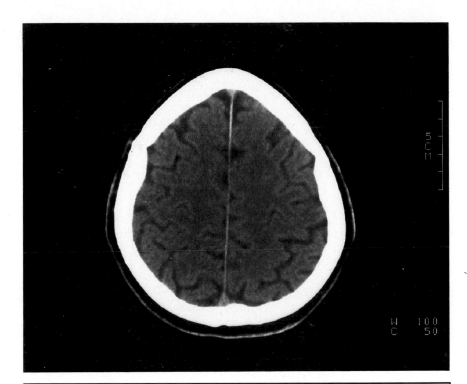

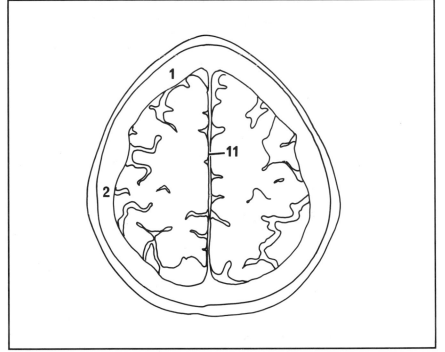

NOTES

This section, through the upper parts of the cerebral hemispheres, gives a clear picture of the distinction between the outer grey matter (12), which contains nerve cells, and the inner white matter (13), made up of nerve fibres. This is in contradistinction to the arrangement of the spinal cord, with the central grey and surrounding white matter.

Note the five layers of the scalp – skin, underlying dense connective tissue (3), the dense epicranial aponeurosis or galea aponeurotica (4), which is separated by a film of loose areolar connective tissue from the outer periosteum of the skull – the pericranium (5). The pericranium is densely adherent to the surface of the skull and passes through the various foramina, where it becomes continuous with the outer endosteal layer of the dura (8). It is also continuous with the sutural ligaments which occupy the cranial sutures.

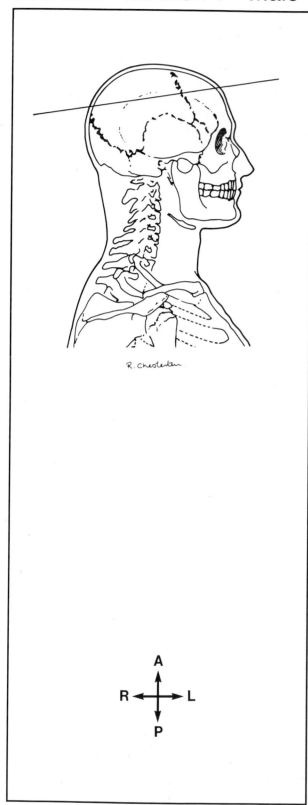

R. Chesterton

A
R — L
P

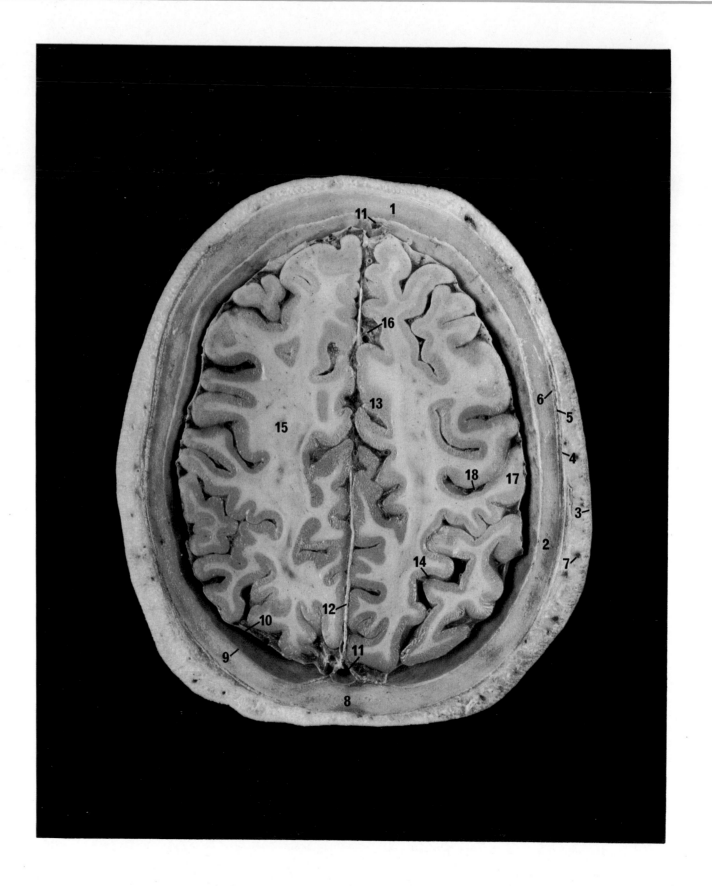

1 Frontal bone
2 Parietal bone
3 Skin and dense subcutaneous tissue
4 Epicranial aponeurosis (galea aponeurotica)
5 Temporalis
6 Pericranium
7 Branch of superficial temporal artery
8 Sagittal suture
9 Dura mater
10 Arachnoid mater
11 Superior sagittal sinus
12 Falx cerebri
13 Cingulate gyrus
14 Parieto-occipital sulcus
15 Corona radiata
16 Anterior cerebral artery (branches)
17 Postcentral gyrus
18 Central sulcus

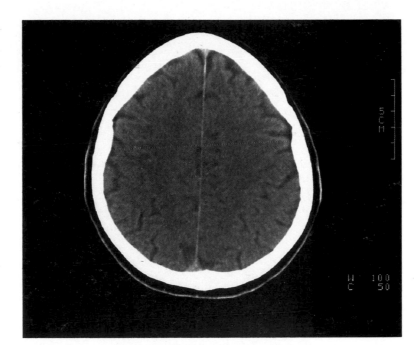

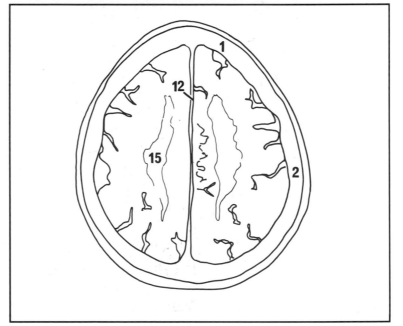

This section allows some of the main gyri and sulci of the cerebrum to be identified. Cross-reference should be made to the photographs of the external aspects and sagittal section of the brain for orientation.

The corona radiata (15) comprises a fan-shaped arrangement of afferent and efferent projection fibres which join the grey matter to lower centres. On the CT image it appears as a curved linear area of low attenuation termed the *centrum semiovale*.

Head – Section 5 – Male

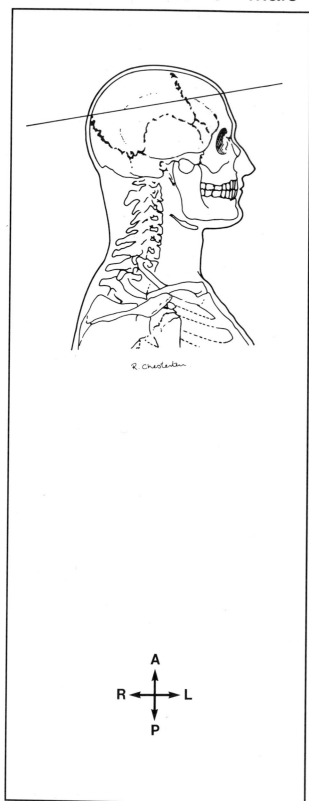

R. Chesterton

A
R ← → L
P

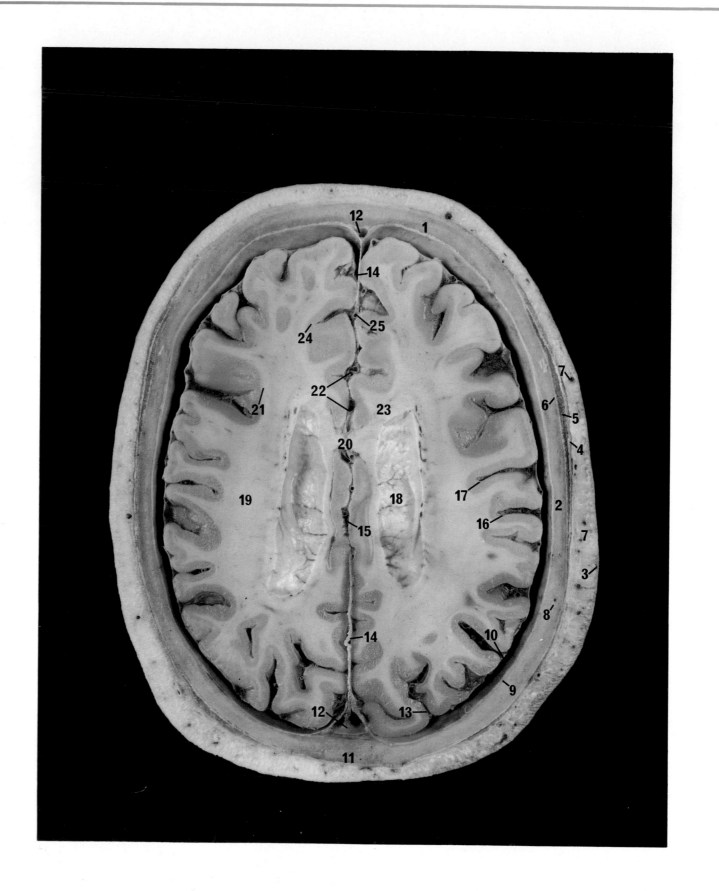

1 Frontal bone
2 Parietal bone
3 Skin and dense subcutaneous tissue
4 Epicranial aponeurosis (galea aponeurotica)
5 Temporalis
6 Pericranium
7 Branches of superficial temporal artery
8 Diploic vein
9 Dura mater
10 Arachnoid mater
11 Sagittal suture
12 Superior sagittal sinus
13 Lunate sulcus
14 Falx cerebri
15 Cingulate gyrus
16 Postcentral sulcus
17 Central sulcus
18 Roof of body of lateral ventricle
19 Corona radiata
20 Corpus callosum
21 Longitudinal fasciculus (corticocortical fibres)
22 Anterior cerebral artery (branches)
23 Forceps minor
24 Cingulate sulcus
25 Inferior sagittal sinus

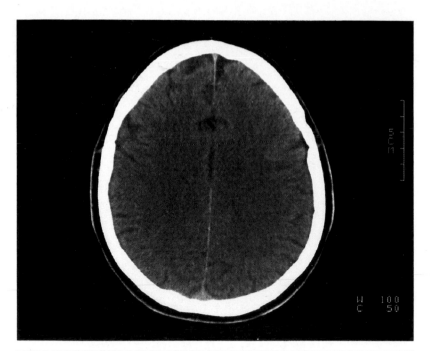

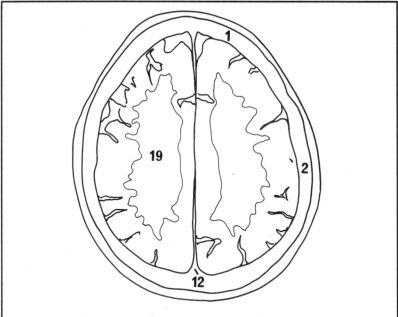

NOTES

This section passes through the roof of the lateral ventricle (18).

The central sulcus, or fissure of Rolando (17), is the most important of the sulcal landmarks, since it separates the pre-central (motor) gyrus from the post-central (sensory) gyrus. It also helps demarcate the frontal and parietal lobes of the cerebrum.

Again the corona radiata (19), or centrum semiovale, is well seen in both the section and CT image.

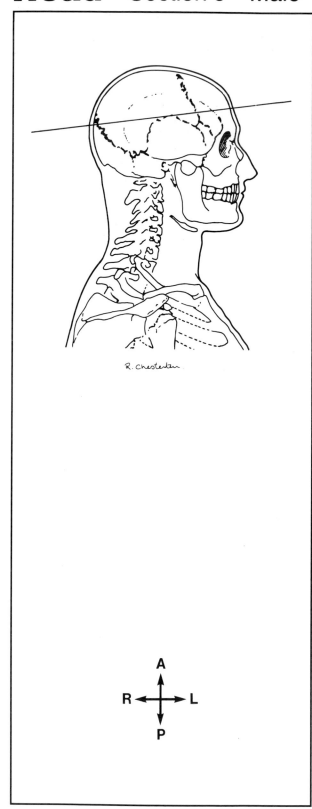

R. Chesterton.

A
R ← → L
P

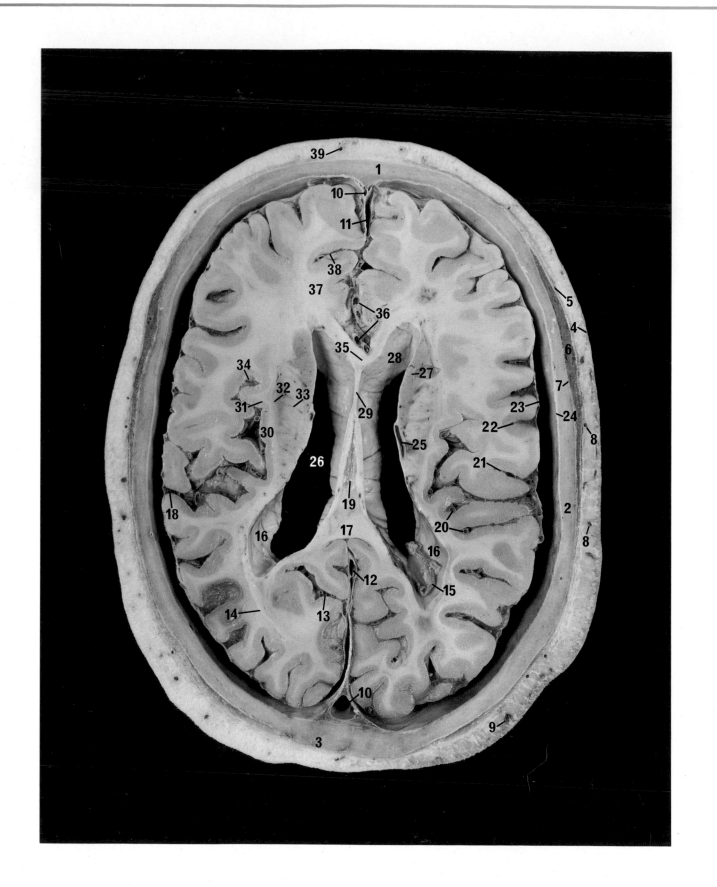

1 Frontal bone
2 Parietal bone
3 Sutural bone
4 Skin and dense subcutaneous tissue
5 Epicranial aponeurosis (galea aponeurotica)
6 Temporalis
7 Pericranium
8 Branches of superficial temporal artery
9 Occipital vein
10 Superior sagittal sinus
11 Falx cerebri
12 Straight sinus
13 Parieto-occipital sulcus
14 Optic radiation
15 Choroid plexus
16 Posterior horn of lateral ventricle
17 Splenium of corpus callosum
18 Lateral sulcus (Sylvian fissure)
19 Third ventricle
20 Middle cerebral artery (branches)
21 Postcentral sulcus
22 Central sulcus
23 Arachnoid mater
24 Dura mater
25 Thalamostriate vein
26 Body of lateral ventricle
27 Body of caudate nucleus
28 Frontal horn of lateral ventricle
29 Septum pellucidum
30 Insula
31 Claustrum
32 Putamen
33 Internal capsule
34 Circular sulcus
35 Genu of corpus callosum
36 Anterior cerebral artery (branches)
37 Forceps minor
38 Cingulate sulcus
39 Supra-orbital artery

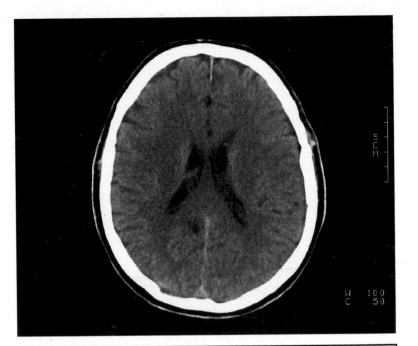

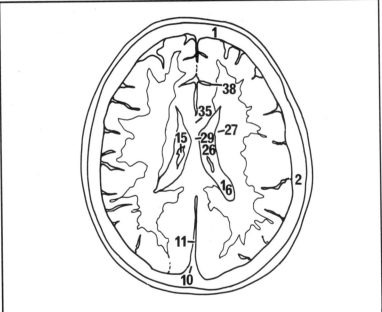

NOTES

This section passes through the bodies of the lateral ventricles (26) and the third ventricle (19).

The lateral ventricles comprise a frontal horn (28) and body (26), which continues with the posterior or occipital horn (16), which, in turn, enters the inferior horn within the temporal lobe. This will be seen in later sections. The lateral ventricles are almost completely separated from each other by the septum pellucidum (29) but communicate indirectly via the third ventricle (19), a narrow slit-like cavity.

The choroid plexuses of the lateral ventricles (15), which are responsible for the production of most of the cerebrospinal fluid (CSF) extend from the inferior horn, through the body to the interventricular foramen where they become continuous with the plexus of the third ventricle.

In addition to the centres of ossification of the named bones of the skull, other centres may occcur in the course of the sutures which give rise to irregular sutural (Wormian) bones (3). They occur most frequently in the region of the lambdoid suture as here, but may sometimes be seen at the anterior, or more especially the posterior, fontanelle. They are usually limited to two or three in number, but may occur in greater numbers in congenital hydrocephalic skulls and other congenital anomalies.

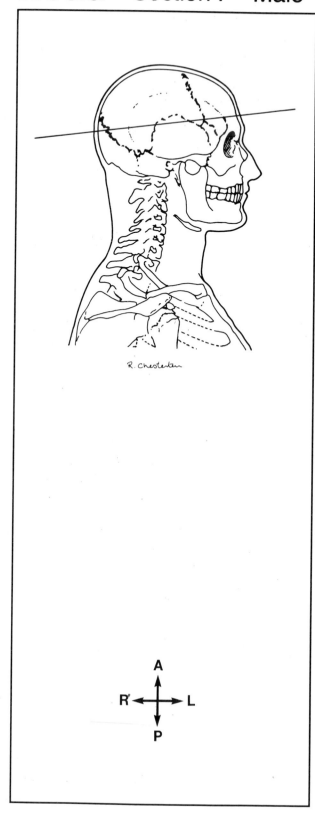

R. Chesterton

A
R ← → L
P

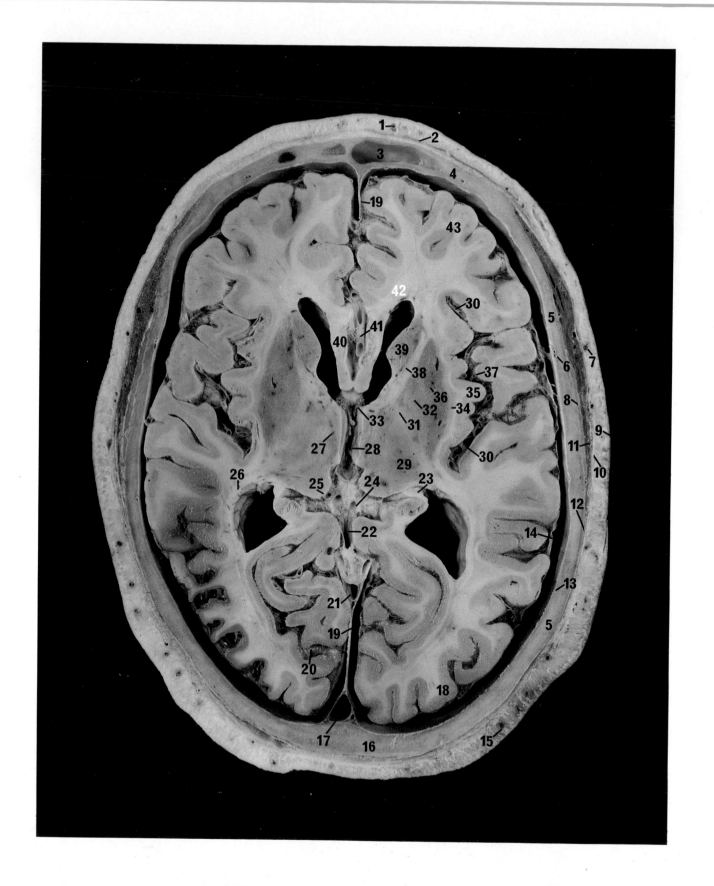

1 Supra-orbital artery	25 Pulvinar of thalamus
2 Frontal belly of occipito-frontalis	26 Optic radiation
3 Frontal sinus	27 Medial nucleus of thalamus
4 Frontal bone	28 Third ventricle
5 Parietal bone	29 Ventroposterior thalamic nucleus
6 Middle meningeal artery and vein	30 Circular sulcus
7 Branch of temporal artery	31 Globus pallidus – internal segment
8 Sliver of squamous part of temporal bone	32 Globus pallidus – external segment
9 Skin and dense sub-cutaneous tissue	33 Choroid plexus in inter-ventricular foramen (Monro)
10 Epicranial aponeurosis (galea aponeurotica)	34 Claustrum
11 Temporalis	35 Insula
12 Pericranium	36 Putamen
13 Dura mater	37 Middle cerebral artery (branches)
14 Arachnoid mater	38 Anterior limb of internal capsule
15 Occipital artery	39 Caudate nucleus – head
16 Squamous part of occipi-tal bone	40 Corpus callosum
17 Superior sagittal sinus	41 Anterior cerebral artery
18 Occipital lobe	42 Frontal horn of lateral ven-tricle
19 Falx cerebri	43 Frontal lobe
20 Calcarine sulcus	
21 Straight sinus	44 Cisterna ambiens
22 Great cerebral vein	45 Cerebellar vermis
23 Fornix	46 Cavum of septum pelluci-dum
24 Internal cerebral vein (branches)	

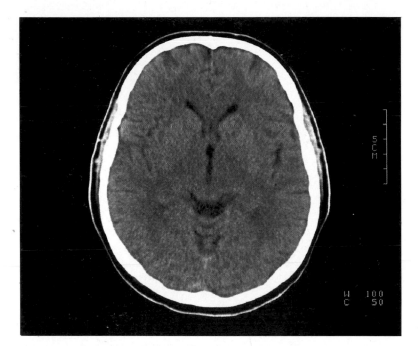

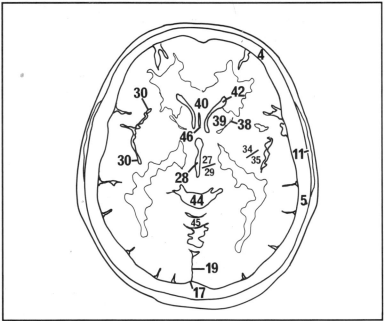

NOTES

This section passes through the apex of the squamous part of the occipital bone (16) and the frontal sinus (3). The latter varies greatly in size from subject to subject, as may be appreciated by the inspection a number of skull radio-graphs.

The interventricular foramen of Munro (33) is well demonstrated and drains the lateral ventricle on both sides into the third ventricle (28), providing a linkage between the ventricular systems within the two cerebral hemispheres.

This section also demonstrates the components of the basal ganglia – the claustrum (34), the lentiform nucleus, made up of the globus pallidus (31, 32) and putamen (36). The latter is largely separated from the head of the caudate nucleus (39) by the anterior limb of the internal capsule (38).

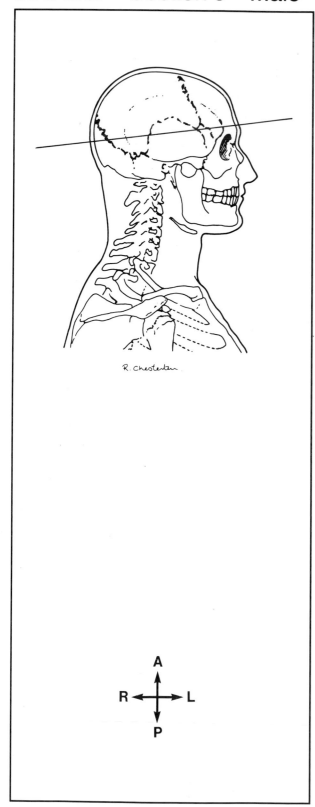

R. Chesterton

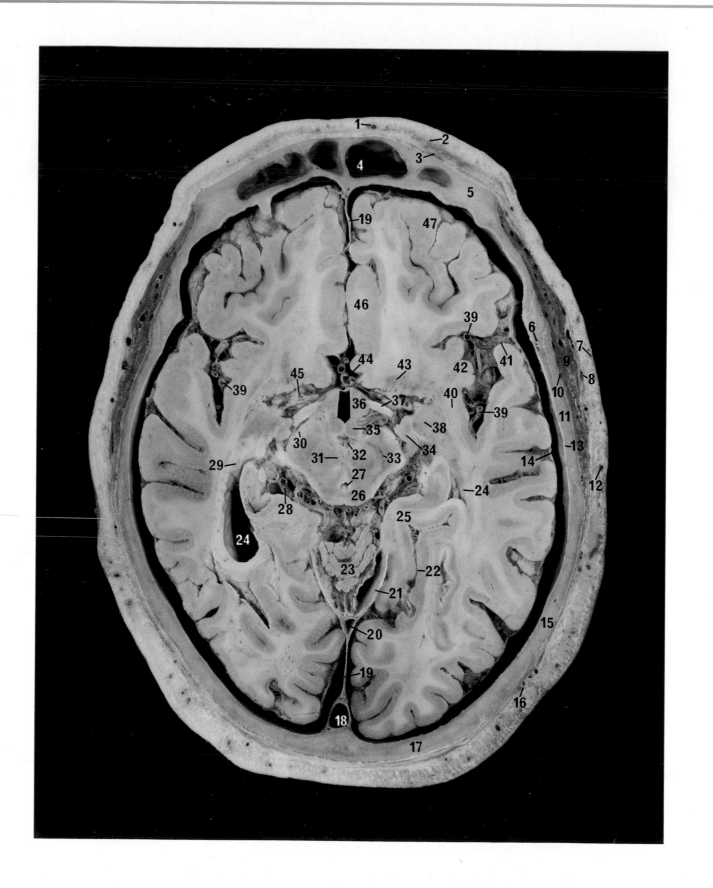

1 Supra-orbital artery	24 Lateral ventricle
2 Orbital part of occipito-frontalis	25 Parahippocampal gyrus
3 Frontal belly of occipito-frontalis	26 Superior colliculus
	27 Aqueduct of Sylvius
4 Frontal sinus	28 Posterior cerebral artery
5 Frontal bone	29 Tail of caudate nucleus
6 Middle meningeal artery and vein	30 Cerebral peduncle
	31 Red nucleus
7 Skin and dense sub-cutaneous tissue	32 Third ventricle
	33 Substantia nigra
8 Epicranial aponeurosis (galea aponeurotica)	34 Cornu ammonis (hippo-campus)
9 Temporalis	35 Mamillary body
10 Pericranium	36 Hypothalamus
11 Squamous part of tem-poral bone	37 Optic tract
	38 Amygdala
12 Superficial temporal artery	39 Middle cerebral artery (branches)
13 Dura mater	40 Claustrum
14 Arachnoid mater	41 Lateral sulcus (Sylvius)
15 Parietal bone	42 Insula
16 Occipital artery	43 Nucleus accumbens septi
17 Squamous part of oc-cipital bone	44 Anterior cerebral artery
	45 Anterior perforated sub-stance
18 Superior sagittal sinus	46 Cingulate gyrus
19 Falx cerebri	47 Orbitofrontal cortex
20 Straight sinus	
21 Tentorium cerebelli	48 Cisterna ambiens
22 Collateral sulcus	49 Temporal lobe
23 Anterior lobe of cerebel-lum	50 Interpeduncular cistern

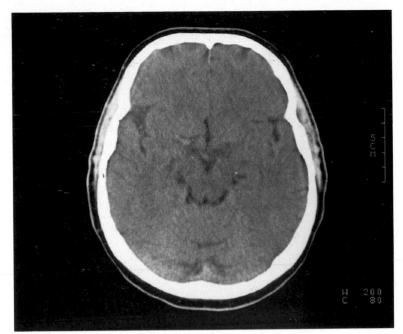

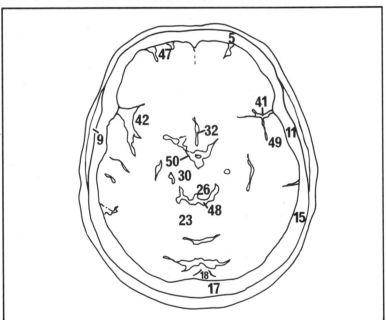

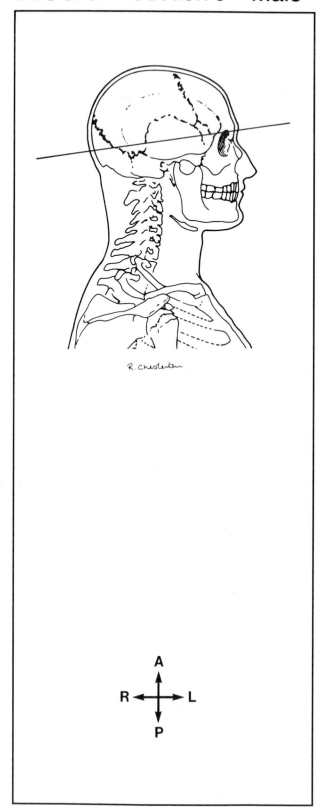

R. Chesterton

A
R ←→ L
P

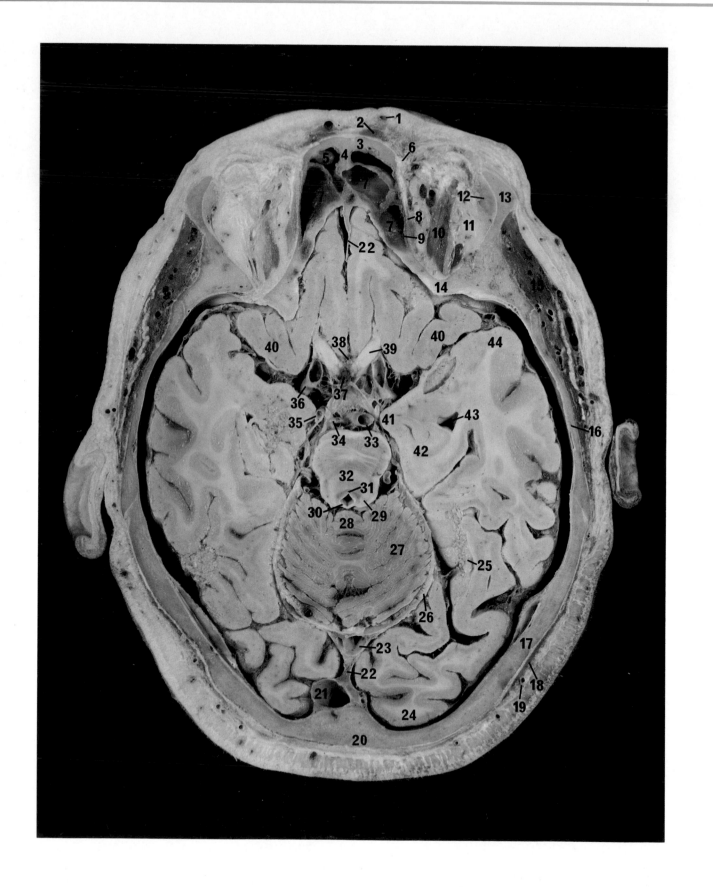

1 Supra-orbital artery
2 Frontal belly of occipito-frontalis
3 Frontal bone
4 Frontal crest
5 Frontal sinus
6 Trochlea
7 Ethmoid air sinuses
8 Superior oblique
9 Orbital plate of ethmoid bone
10 Superior rectus underlying levator palpebri superioris
11 Orbital fat
12 Lacrimal gland
13 Zygomatic process of frontal bone
14 Lesser wing of sphenoid bone
15 Temporalis
16 Temporal bone
17 Parietal bone
18 Posterior belly of occipito-frontalis
19 Occipital artery
20 Occipital bone
21 Superior sagittal sinus
22 Falx cerebri
23 Straight sinus
24 Occipital pole
25 Floor of lateral ventricle (occipital horn)

26 Tentorium cerebelli (outer edge)
27 Anterior lobe of cerebellum
28 Cerebellar vermis
29 Inferior colliculus
30 Aqueduct of Sylvius
31 Locus coeruleus
32 Decussation of superior cerebellar peduncle
33 Basilar artery
34 Superior cerebellar artery
35 Posterior cerebral artery
36 Internal carotid artery
37 Pituitary infundibulum
38 Optic chiasma
39 Optic nerve (II)
40 Orbitofrontal cortex
41 Uncus of parahippo-campal gyrus
42 Hippocampus
43 Temporal horn of lateral ventricle
44 Temporal pole

45 Posterior clinoid process
46 Anterior clinoid process
47 Mastoid air cells
48 Petrous temporal bone
49 Pons
50 Fourth ventricle

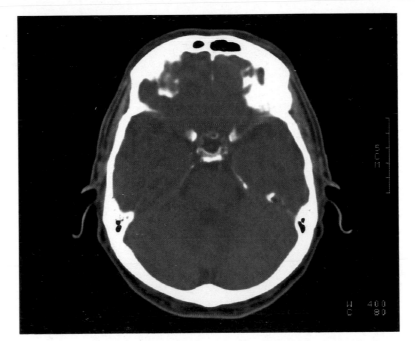

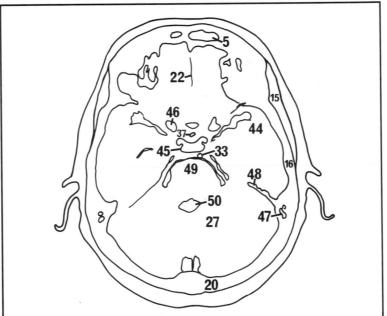

NOTES

This section traverses the upper part of the orbits, the mid brain at the level of the inferior colliculus (29) and the anterior lobe of the cerebellum (27).

The straight sinus (23) lies in the sagittal plane of the tentorium cerebelli (26) at its attachment to the falx cerebri (22). It receives both the inferior sagittal sinus and the great cerebral vein, and drains posteriorly, usually into the left but occasionally into the right, transverse sinus.

The clinoid processes (45, 46) are well seen on the CT image. The anterior clinoid processes arise from the lesser wing of the sphenoid (see section 14); the posterior processes are the postero-lateral margins of the dorsum sellae.

Head – Section 10 – Male

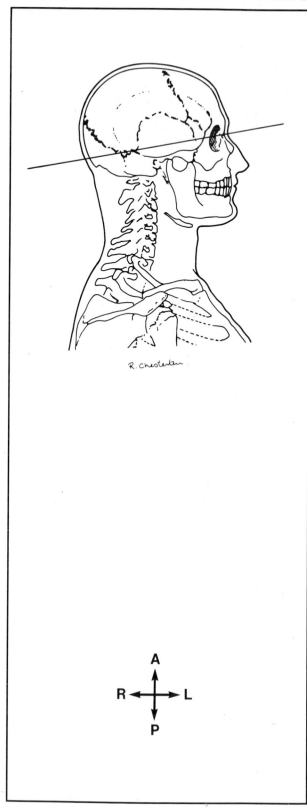

R. Chesterton

A
R ←→ L
P

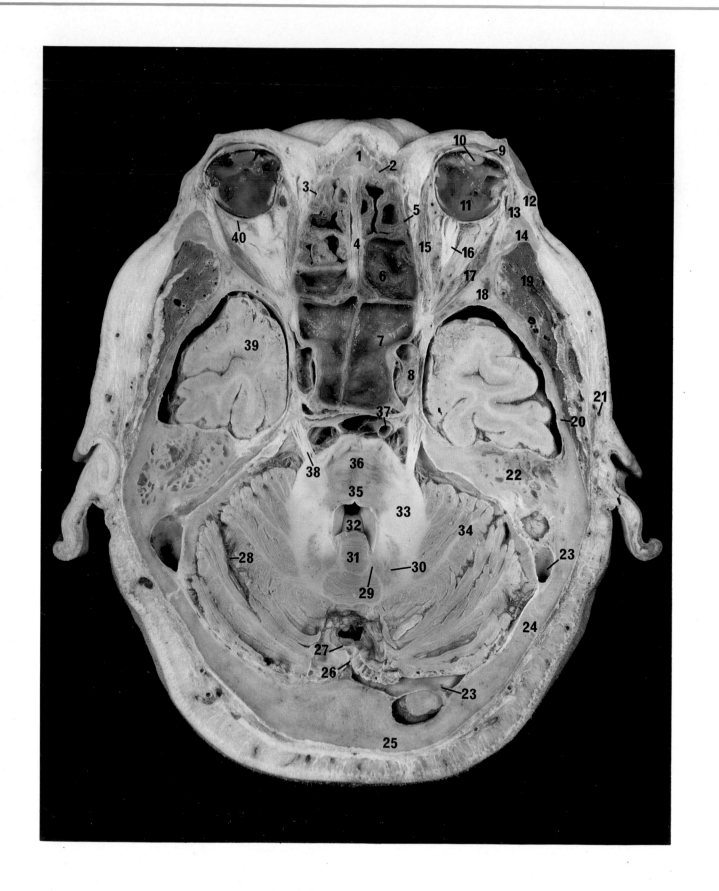

1 Nasal bone
2 Frontal process of maxilla
3 Nasolacrimal duct
4 Perpendicular plate of ethmoid bone
5 Orbital plate of ethmoid bone
6 Posterior ethmoidal air cells
7 Sphenoidal sinus
8 Internal carotid artery within cavernous sinus
9 Cornea
10 Lens
11 Vitreous humour
12 Orbicularis oculi – orbital part
13 Orbicularis oculi – palpebral part
14 Frontal process of zygomatic bone
15 Medial rectus
16 Optic nerve (II)
17 Lateral rectus
18 Greater wing of sphenoid bone
19 Temporalis
20 Squamous part of temporal bone
21 Superficial temporal artery and vein

22 Mastoid air cells
23 Transverse sinus
24 Parietal bone
25 Squamous part of occipital bone
26 Falx cerebelli
27 Superior sagittal sinus
28 Posterolateral fissure
29 Emboliform (interposed) nucleus
30 Dentate nucleus
31 Vermis of cerebellum
32 Fourth ventricle
33 Middle cerebellar peduncle
34 Hemisphere of cerebellum
35 Pontine tegmentum
36 Pontine nuclei
37 Basilar artery
38 Trigeminal nerve (V)
39 Temporal lobe
40 Sclera

41 Crista galli of ethmoid
42 Petrous part of temporal bone
43 Internal auditory meatus

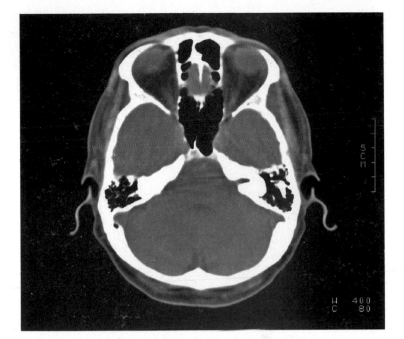

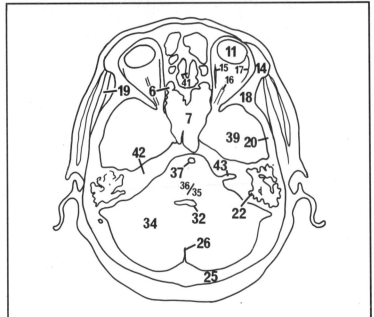

NOTES

This section transects the eyeballs, the sphenoidal sinus (7) and the pons (36) at the level of the middle cerebellar peduncles (33).

The structure of the orbit in horizontal section can be appreciated in this section. The eyeball with its cornea (9), lens (10) and vitreous humour (11) contained within the tough sclera (40), and the optic nerve (16) lie surrounded by the extrinsic muscles (15, 17). The slit-like nasolacrimal duct (3) drains downwards into the inferior meatus.

The fourth ventricle (32) lies above the tegmentum of the pons (35) and below the vermis of the cerebellum (31).

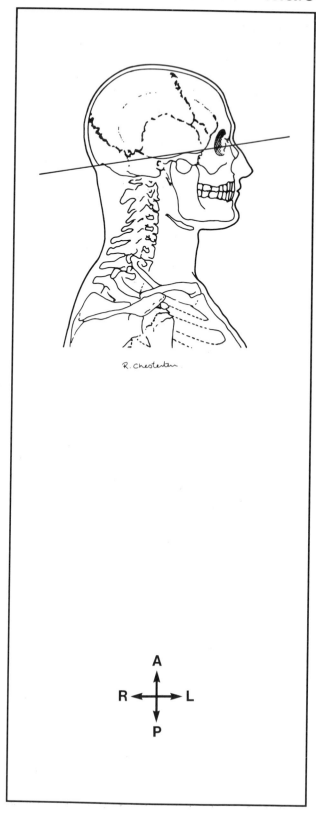

R. Chesterton

A
R ← → L
P

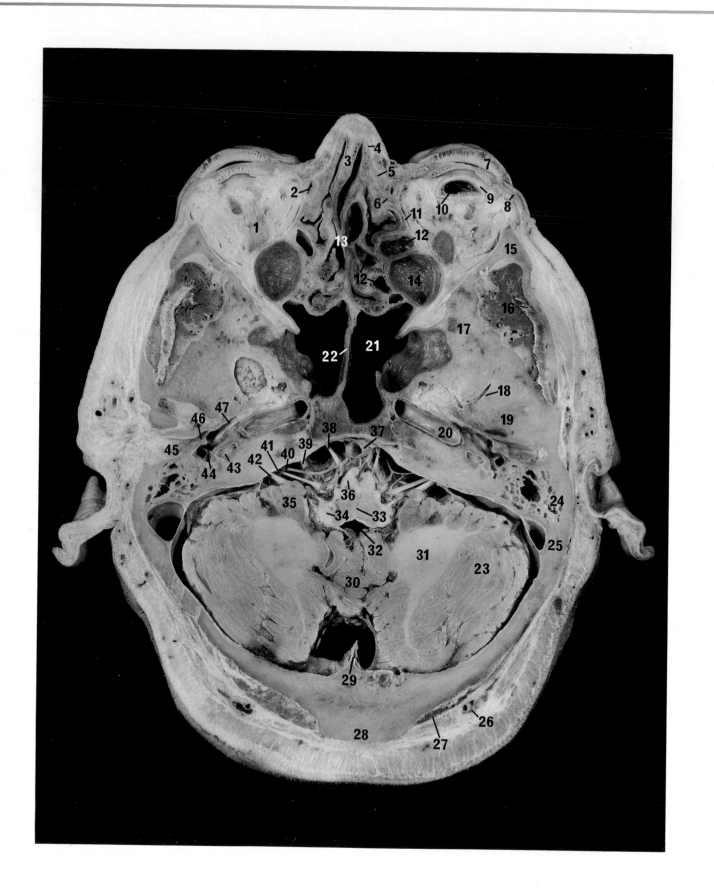

1 Inferior rectus
2 Nasolacrimal duct
3 Cartilage of nasal septum
4 Nasal bone
5 Frontal process of maxilla
6 Lacrimal bone
7 Upper eyelid
8 Orbicularis oculi
9 Sclera
10 Vitreous humour
11 Orbital plate of ethmoid bone
12 Ethmoid air cells
13 Perpendicular plate of ethmoid bone
14 Apex of maxillary antrum
15 Frontal process of zygomatic bone
16 Temporalis
17 Greater wing of sphenoid bone
18 Middle meningeal artery
19 Petrous part of temporal bone
20 Internal carotid artery
21 Sphenoidal sinus
22 Septum of sphenoidal sinus
23 Cerebellar hemisphere
24 Mastoid air cells
25 Transverse sinus
26 Occipital artery and vein
27 Trapezius

28 External occipital protruberance
29 Falx cerebelli
30 Vermis
31 Middle cerebellar peduncle
32 Fourth ventricle with choroid plexus
33 Medulla oblongata
34 Inferior cerebellar peduncle
35 Flocculus
36 Pyramidal tract
37 Basilar artery
38 Abducent nerve (VI)
39 Trigeminal nerve (V)
40 Labyrinthine artery
41 Facial nerve (VII)
42 Vestibulocochlear (auditory) nerve (VIII)
43 Cochlea
44 Stapes
45 External auditory meatus
46 Tympanic membrane and handle of malleus
47 Auditory tube (eustachian)

48 Lens
49 Medial rectus
50 Lateral rectus
51 Foramen rotundum

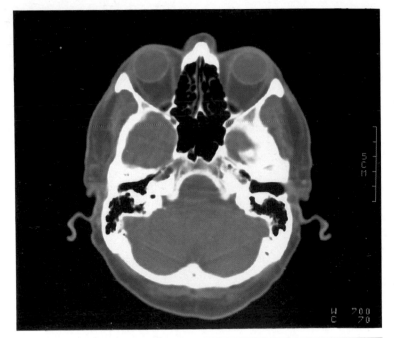

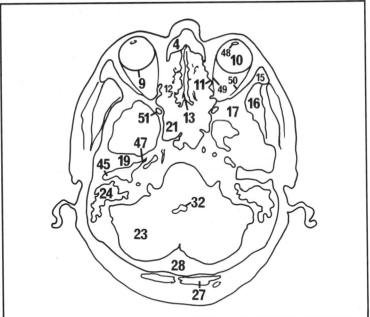

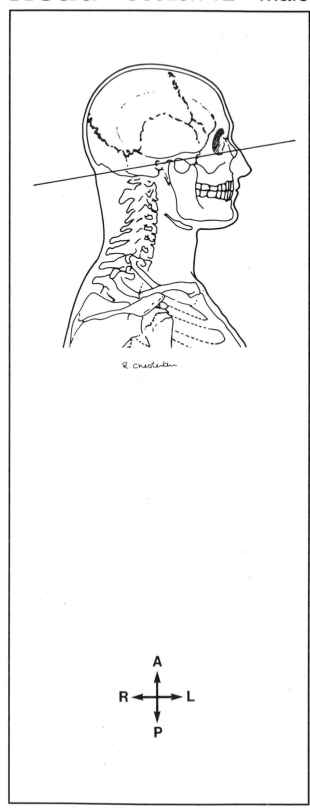

R. Chesterton

A
R ← → L
P

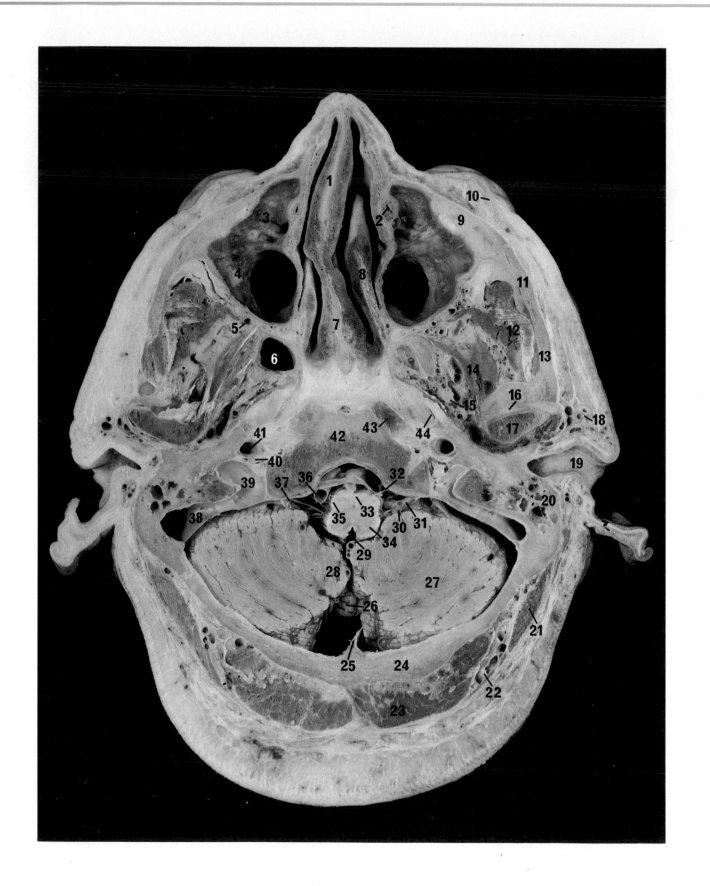

1 Cartilage of nasal septum	26 Vermis
2 Nasolacrimal duct	27 Cerebellar hemisphere
3 Orifice of maxillary sinus	28 Tonsil of cerebellum
4 Maxillary sinus	29 Fourth ventricle (median aperture of roof)
5 Maxillary artery	30 Anterior inferior cerebellar artery
6 Sphenoidal sinus	31 Glossopharyngeal nerve (IX)
7 Vomer	32 Hypoglossal nerve (XII)
8 Middle nasal concha	33 Pyramidal tract
9 Maxilla	34 Medulla
10 Orbicularis oculi	35 Inferior olive
11 Zygomatic bone	36 Vertebral artery
12 Temporalis and tendon	37 Vagus nerve (X)
13 Zygomatic process of temporal bone	38 Sigmoid sinus
14 Lateral pterygoid	39 Bulb of internal jugular vein
15 Trigeminal nerve (V)	40 Glossopharyngeal nerve, vagus nerve, and accessory nerve (IX, X and XI)
16 Articular disc of temporomandibular joint	41 Internal carotid artery
17 Head of mandible	42 Basi-occiput
18 Superficial temporal artery and vein	43 Longus capitis
19 External auditory meatus	44 Auditory (eustachian) tube
20 Mastoid air cells	
21 Sternocleidomastoid	45 Pterygopalatine fossa (apex)
22 Occipital artery and vein	46 Foramen ovale
23 Trapezius	
24 Occipital bone – squamous part	
25 Falx cerebelli	

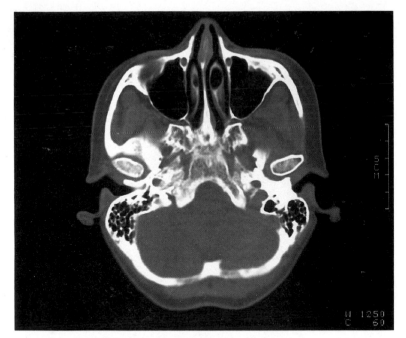

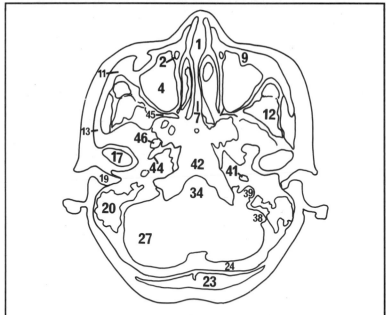

NOTES

This section transects the maxillary sinus (4) and the basiocciput (42) and passes through the external auditory meatus (19).

At this level the vertebral arteries (36) are running cranially from their entry into the skull at the foramen magnum to form the basilar artery.

The sigmoid sinus (38) runs forward to emerge from the skull at the jugular foramen, at which it becomes the bulb of the internal jugular vein (39). Exiting through the jugular foramen anterior to the vein lie, from anterior to posterior, the glossopharyngeal, vagus and accessory cranial nerves (40).

The maxillary nerve (V^{ii}) passes into the pterygopalatine fossa (45 on this CT image), having traversed the foramen rotundum (see CT image, section 11). The mandibular nerve (V^{iii}) leaves the skull via the foramen ovale (46).

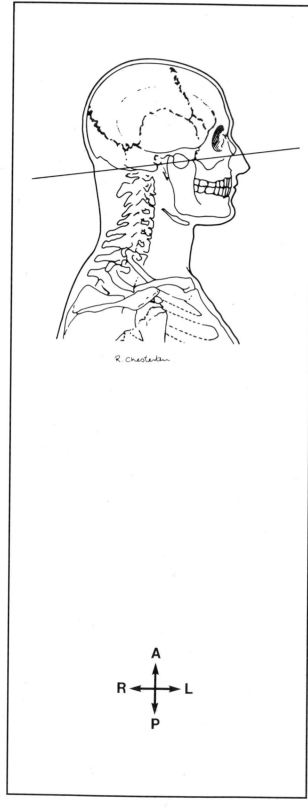

R. Chesterton

A
R ← → L
P

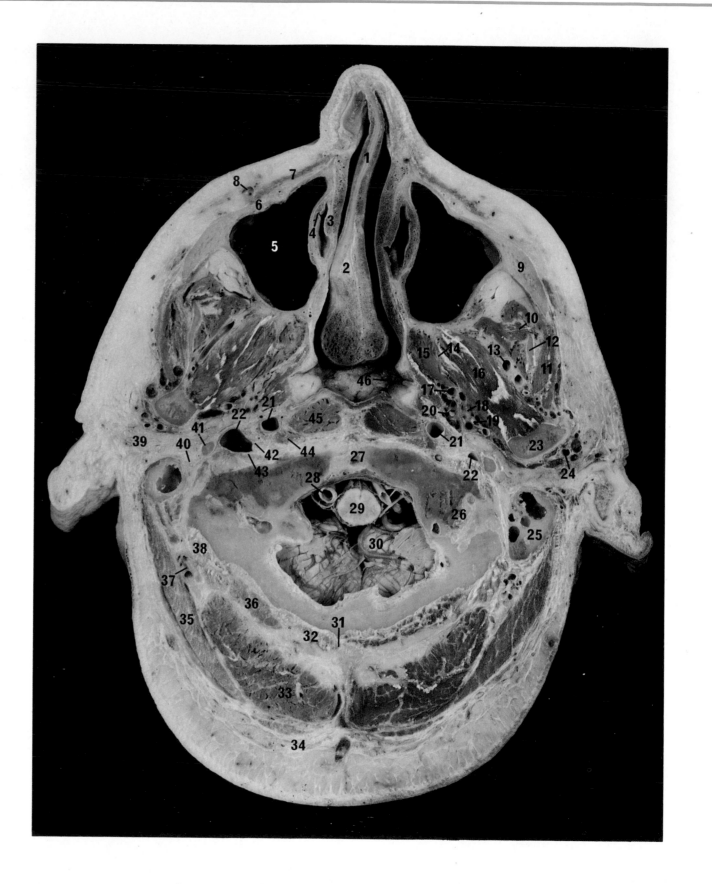

1 Cartilage of nasal septum	26 Base of occipital condyle
2 Vomer	27 Basilar part of occipital bone
3 Inferior nasal concha	28 Vertebral artery
4 Orifice of nasolacrimal duct	29 Spinal cord
5 Maxillary sinus	30 Tonsil of cerebellum
6 Maxilla	31 External occipital crest
7 Levator labii superioris	32 Rectus capitis posterior minor
8 Facial vein	33 Semispinalis capitis
9 Zygomatic bone	34 Trapezius
10 Tendon of temporalis	35 Sternocleidomastoid
11 Masseter	36 Rectus capitis posterior major
12 Coronoid process of mandible	37 Occipital artery and vein
13 Maxillary artery and vein	38 Obliquus capitis superior
14 Lateral pterygoid plate of sphenoid	39 Parotid gland
15 Medial pterygoid	40 Facial nerve (VII)
16 Lateral pterygoid	41 Styloid process
17 Pterygoid artery and pterygoid venous plexus	42 Glossopharyngeal nerve (IX), vagus nerve (X) and accessory nerve (XI)
18 Lingual nerve (V^{III})	43 Hypoglossal nerve (XII)
19 Inferior alveolar nerve (V^{III})	44 Rectus capitis anterior
20 Chorda tympani	45 Longus capitis
21 Internal carotid artery	46 Opening of auditory (eustachian) tube
22 Internal jugular vein	
23 Head of mandible	
24 Superficial temporal artery	47 Nasopharynx
25 Mastoid air cells	48 Parapharyngeal space
	49 Pharyngeal recess

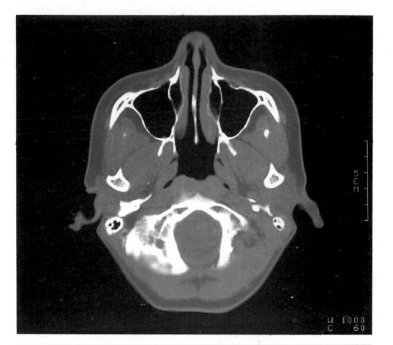

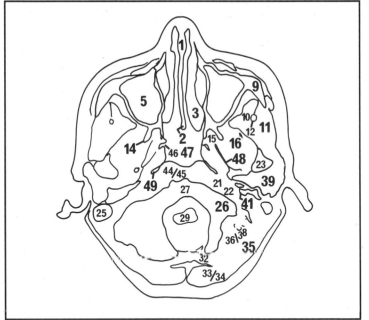

NOTES

This section traverses the nasal septum (1) at the level of the inferior nasal concha (3), beneath which opens the nasolacrimal duct (4). Posteriorly the plane passes through the uppermost part of the spinal cord (29) and the cerebellar tonsil (30).

The internal jugular vein (22) in this specimen is small, especially on the left side. The chorda tympani (20) is seen here as it emerges from the petro-tympanic fissure to join the lingual nerve (18) about 2 cm below the base of the skull. It subserves taste sensation to the anterior two-thirds of the tongue as well as supplying secretomotor fibres to the submandibular and sublingual salivary glands.

The tonsil of the cerebellum (30), on the inferior aspect of the cerebellar hemisphere, lies immediately above the foramen magnum. Withdrawal of CSF at lumbar puncture in a patient with raised intracranial pressure is dangerous as it may result in lethal herniation of the tonsils through this bony ring.

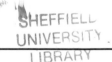

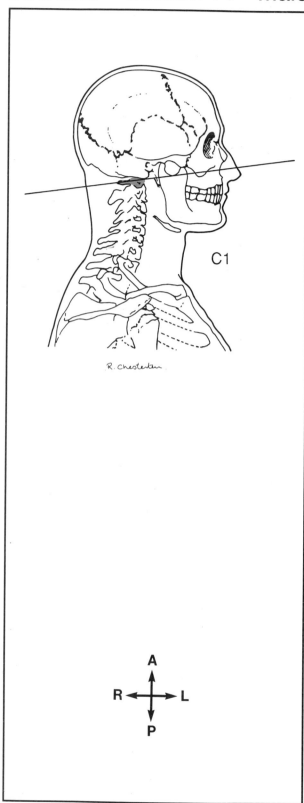

C1

R. Chesterton

A
R — L
P

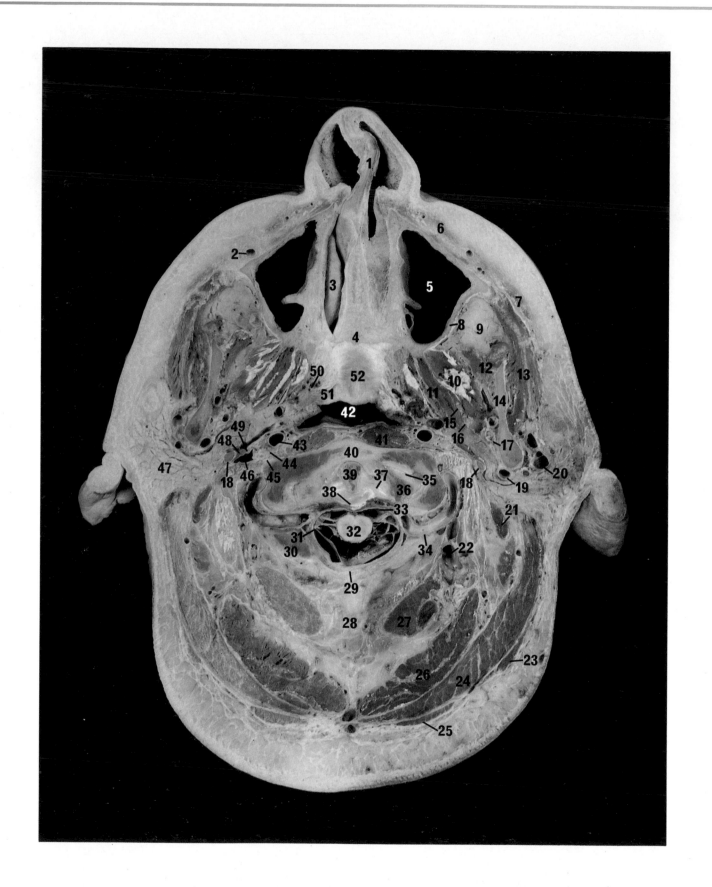

1 Cartilage of nasal septum	30 Posterior arch of atlas
2 Facial vein	31 Spinal root of accessory nerve (XI)
3 Inferior nasal concha	32 Spinal cord within dural sheath
4 Horizontal plate of palatine bone	33 Membrana tectoria
5 Maxillary sinus	34 Vertebral artery
6 Levator labii superioris	35 Atlanto-occipital joint
7 Zygomaticus major	36 Condyle of occipital bone
8 Maxilla	37 Alar ligament
9 Buccal fat pad	38 Transverse ligament of atlas (first cervical vertebra)
10 Lateral pterygoid	39 Dens of axis (odontoid process of second cervical vertebra)
11 Medial pterygoid	
12 Temporalis	
13 Masseter	40 Anterior arch of atlas (first cervical vertebra)
14 Ramus of mandible	41 Longus capitis
15 Lingual nerve (V^{III})	42 Nasopharynx
16 Inferior alveolar artery vein and nerve (V^{III})	43 Internal carotid artery
17 Maxillary artery	44 Glossopharyngeal nerve (IX), vagus nerve (X)
18 Styloid process	45 Sympathetic chain
19 External carotid artery	46 Internal jugular vein
20 Retromandibular vein	47 Parotid gland
21 Posterior belly of digastric	48 Stylopharyngeus
22 Vertebral vein	49 Accessory nerve (XI)
23 Sternocleidomastoid	50 Pterygoid venous plexus
24 Splenius	51 Tensor veli palatini
25 Trapezius	52 Soft palate
26 Semispinalis capitis	
27 Rectus capitis posterior major	53 Pharyngeal recess
28 Ligamentum nuchae	54 Parapharyngeal space
29 Posterior atlanto-occipital membrane	

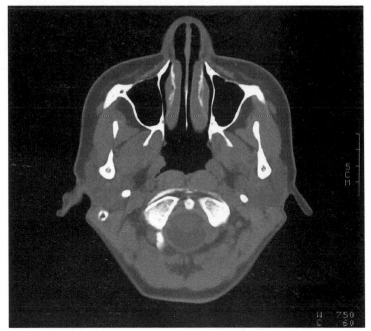

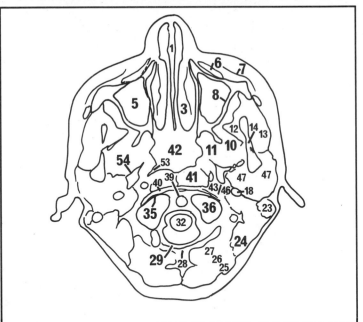

NOTES

This section traverses the nasal cavity through its inferior meatus below the inferior concha (3), the hard palate at the horizontal plate of the palatine bone (4) and the tip of the dens of the axis, the second cervical vertebra (39).

The external carotid artery (19) divides at the neck of the mandible into the superficial temporal artery and the maxillary artery (17).

Note that the outer endosteal layer of the dura mater of the skull blends with the pericranium at the foramen magnum. The dural sheath surrounding the spinal cord (32) represents the continuation of the inner meningeal layer of the cerebral dura (see section 1).

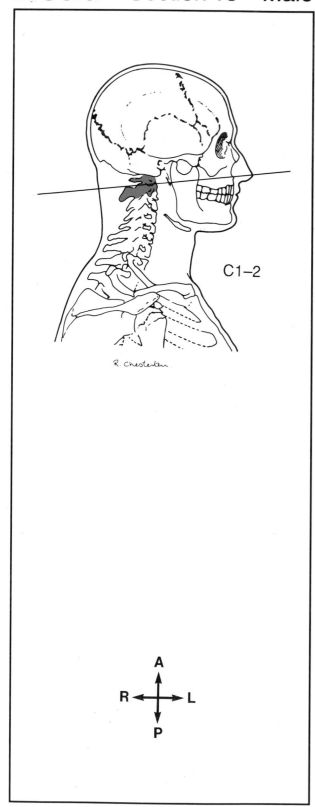

C1–2

R. Chesterton

A
R ← → L
P

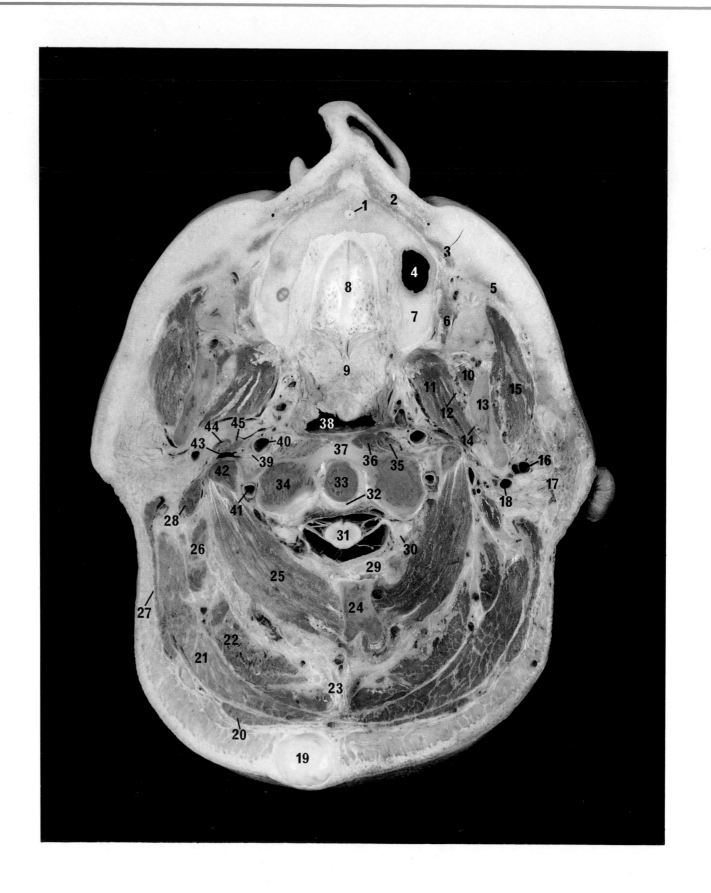

1 Nasopalatine nerve (V^ii) within incisive canal
2 Orbicularis oris
3 Levator angulis oris
4 Maxillary antrum
5 Zygomaticus major
6 Buccinator
7 Alveolar process of maxilla
8 Hard palate
9 Soft palate
10 Temporalis
11 Medial pterygoid
12 Lingual nerve (V^iii)
13 Ramus of mandible
14 Inferior alveolar artery, vein and nerve
15 Masseter
16 Retromandibular vein
17 Parotid gland
18 External carotid artery
19 Dermoid cyst of scalp
20 Trapezius
21 Splenius capitis
22 Semispinalis capitis
23 Ligamentum nuchae
24 Spine of axis (second cervical vertebra)
25 Obliquus capitis inferior
26 Longissimus capitis
27 Sternocleidomastoid
28 Posterior belly of digastric
29 Posterior arch of atlas (first cervical vertebra)

30 Dorsal root ganglion of second cervical nerve
31 Spinal cord within dural sheath
32 Transverse ligament of atlas
33 Dens of axis (odontoid process of second cervical vertebra)
34 Lateral mass of atlas (first cervical vertebra)
35 Longus capitis
36 Longus colli
37 Anterior arch of atlas (first cervical vertebra)
38 Nasopharynx
39 Vagus nerve (X) and hypoglossal nerve (XII)
40 Internal carotid artery
41 Vertebral artery
42 Transverse process of atlas (first cervical vertebra)
43 Internal jugular vein
44 Styloid process with origins of styloglossus and stylohyoid and glossopharyngeal nerve (IX)
45 Stylopharyngeus

46 Levator and tensor veli palatini
47 Parapharyngeal space
48 Inferior nasal concha
49 Cartilage of nasal septum

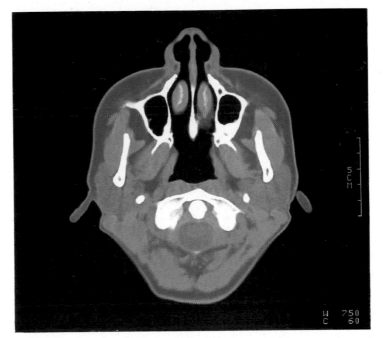

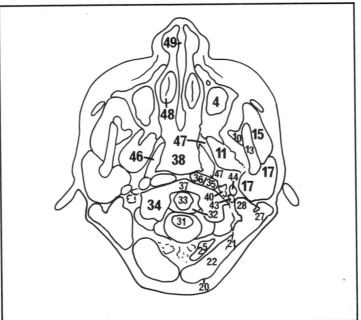

NOTES

This section traverses the hard and soft palate (8, 9), the nasopharynx (38), the dens (33) and the spine of the axis (24). The CT image is rather more cranial.

Flexion and extension of the skull (nodding movements of the head) take place at the atlanto-occipital joint between the upper facet of the lateral mass of the atlas (34) and the corresponding facet on the occipital bone. Rotation of the skull (looking to the left and right) takes place at the atlanto-axial articulation between the dens (33) and the facet on the anterior arch of the atlas (37). The transverse ligament of the atlas (32) is dense and is the principal structure in preventing posterior dislocation of the dens.

The obliquus capitis inferior (25) forms the lower outer limb of the sub-occipital triangle. The vertebral artery (41), on emerging from the foramen transversarium of the atlas, enters this triangle on its ascending course to the foramen magnum.

Note that this subject has a large dermoid cyst of the scalp (19).

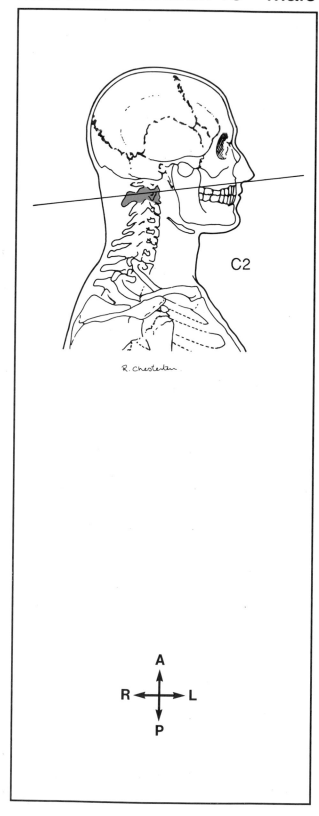

C2

R. Chesterton

A
R ← → L
P

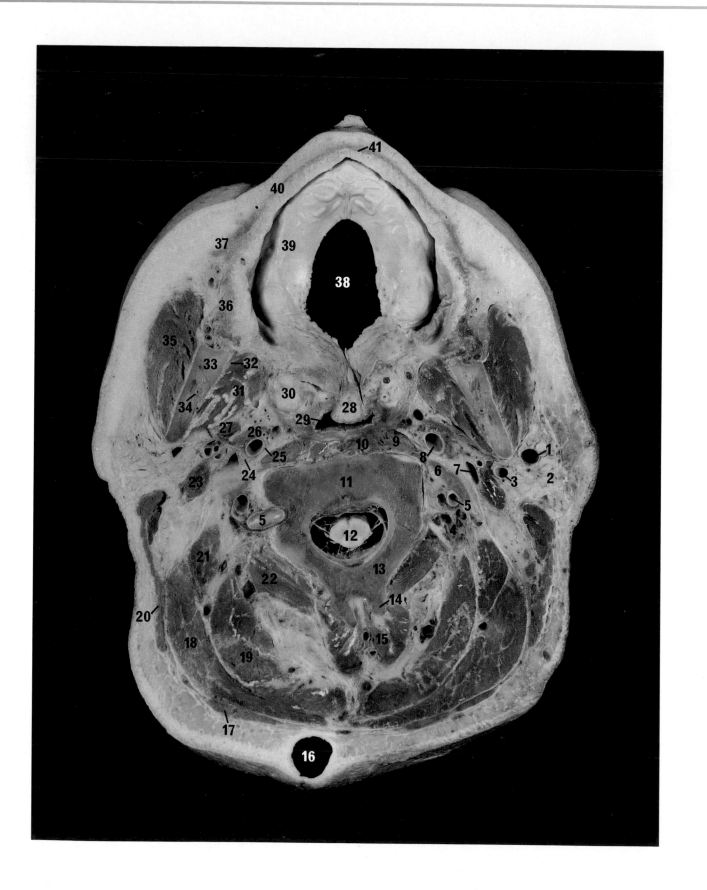

1 Retromandibular vein
2 Parotid gland
3 External carotid artery
4 Vertebral vein
5 Vertebral artery
6 Scalenus medius
7 Internal jugular vein
8 Internal carotid artery
9 Longus capitis
10 Longus colli
11 Body of axis (second cervical vertebra)
12 Spinal cord within dural sheath
13 Lamina of axis (second cervical vertebra)
14 Spine of axis (second cervical vertebra)
15 Semispinalis cervicis
16 Dermoid cyst of scalp
17 Trapezius
18 Splenius
19 Semispinalis capitis
20 Sternocleidomastoid
21 Longissimus capitis
22 Obliquus capitis inferior
23 Posterior belly of digastric
24 Vagus nerve (X) and hypoglossal nerve (XII)
25 Sympathetic chain
26 Stylopharyngeus and glossopharyngeal nerve (IX)

27 Styloglossus and stylohyoid (posteriorly)
28 Base of uvula
29 Nasopharynx
30 Palatine tonsil
31 Medial pterygoid
32 Lingual nerve (V^{III})
33 Ramus of mandible
34 Inferior alveolar artery, vein and nerve (V^{III}) within mandibular canal
35 Masseter
36 Buccinator
37 Levator anguli oris
38 Mouth
39 Alveolar margin
40 Orbicularis oris
41 Mucous gland of lip

42 Hard palate
43 Soft palate
44 Styloid process
45 Parapharyngeal space
46 Anterior arch of atlas
47 Dens of axis (odontoid process of second cervical vertebra)
48 Posterior arch of atlas (first cervical vetebra)
49 Foramen transversarium

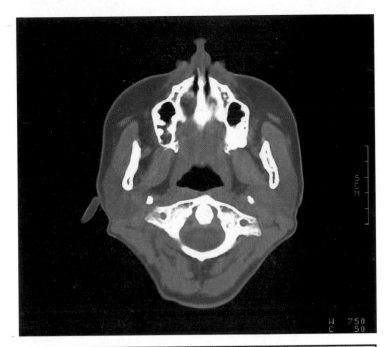

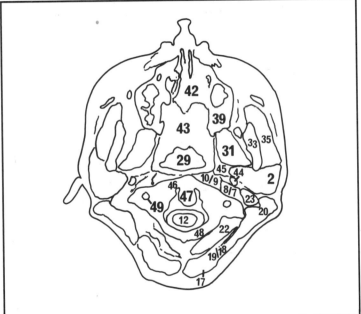

NOTES

This section passes through the alveolar margin (39) of the upper jaw and through the body of the axis (11). The CT image is at a more cranial level.

The vertebral artery (5) on the right side of this specimen is tortuous and bulges laterally between the transverse processes of the atlas and axis, a not uncommon feature in arteriosclerotic subjects. Each cervical vertebra bears its characteristic foramen transversarium (49) within its transverse process. The vertebral artery, with its accompanying vein, ascends through the foramina of C6 to C1 to gain access to the foramen magnum.

The lips are lined by mucous membrane enclosing the orbicularis oris (40), the labial vessels and nerves, fibrofatty connective tissue and the labial mucous glands (41). These glands lie between the mucosa and underlying muscle, are about 0.5 cm in diameter and resemble mucous salivary glands. Their ducts drain into the vestibule of the mouth. These glands, like those studded over the oral aspect of the palate, are occasional sites of pleomorphic adenomas, which are similar to those more commonly seen in the parotid gland.

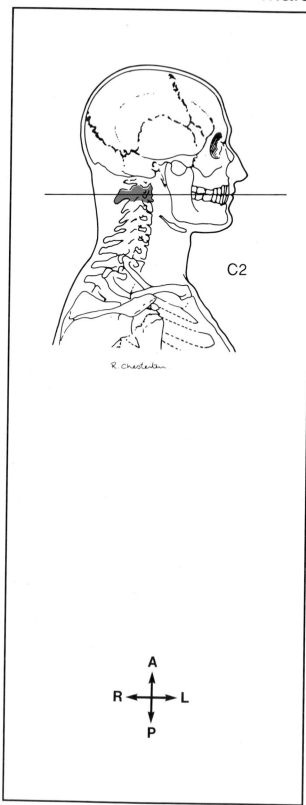

C2

R. Chesterton

A
R ← → L
P

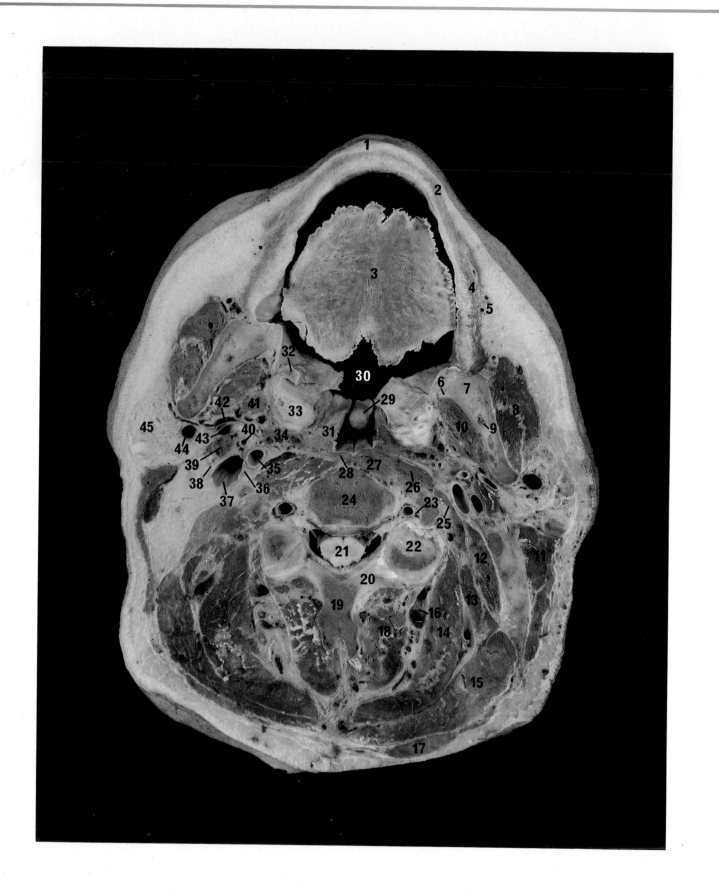

1 Upper lip
2 Orbicularis oris
3 Tongue
4 Buccinator
5 Facial artery and vein
6 Lingual nerve (V^{III})
7 Ramus of mandible
8 Masseter
9 Inferior alveolar artery, vein and nerve (V^{III}) within mandibular canal
10 Medial pterygoid
11 Sternocleidomastoid
12 Levator scapulae
13 Longissimus capitis
14 Semispinalis capitis
15 Splenius
16 Deep cervical vein
17 Trapezius
18 Semispinalis cervicis
19 Spine of axis (second cervical vertebra)
20 Lamina of axis (second cervical vertebra)
21 Spinal cord within dural sheath
22 Superior articular process of axis (second cervical vertebra)
23 Vertebral artery and vein
24 Body of axis (second cervical vertebra)

25 Scalenus medius
26 Longus capitis
27 Longus colli
28 Constrictor muscle of pharynx
29 Uvula
30 Oropharynx
31 Palatopharyngeal arch with palatopharyngeus
32 Palatoglossal arch with palatoglossus
33 Palatine tonsil
34 Stylopharyngeus
35 Internal carotid artery
36 Vagus nerve (X)
37 Internal jugular vein
38 Accessory nerve (XI)
39 Digastric (posterior belly)
40 External carotid artery
41 Styloglossus
42 Stylohyoid
43 Posterior auricular artery
44 Retromandibular vein
45 Parotid gland

46 Nasopharynx
47 Parapharyngeal space
48 Alveolar process of maxilla

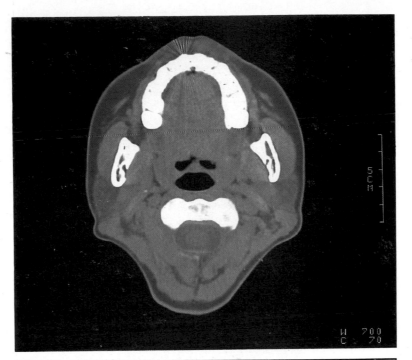

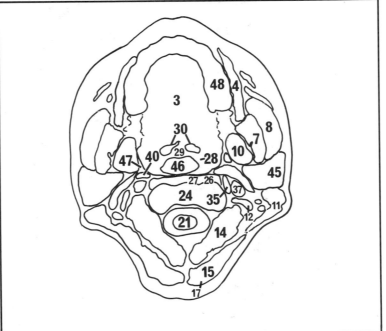

This section traverses the upper lip (1), the tongue (3), the uvula (29) and the axis (19, 20, 22, 24). The plane of the CT image is slightly more cranial.

The palatine tonsil (33) lies in the tonsillar fossa between the anterior and posterior pillars of the fauces. The anterior pillar, or palatoglossal arch (32), forms the boundary between the buccal cavity and the oropharynx (30). It fuses with the lateral wall of the tongue and contains the palatoglossus muscle. The posterior pillar, or palatopharyngeal arch (31), blends with the wall of the pharynx and contains the palatopharyngeus muscle.

The tonsil consists of a collection of lymphoid tissue covered by a squamous epithelium; a unique histological combination which makes it easy to identify under the microscope. From late puberty onwards the lymphoid tissue undergoes progressive atrophy.

The prominent deep cervical vein (16) is a useful landmark in separating the deeply placed semispinalis cervicis muscle (18) from the more superficially placed semispinalis capitis (14); this is seen again in section 18.

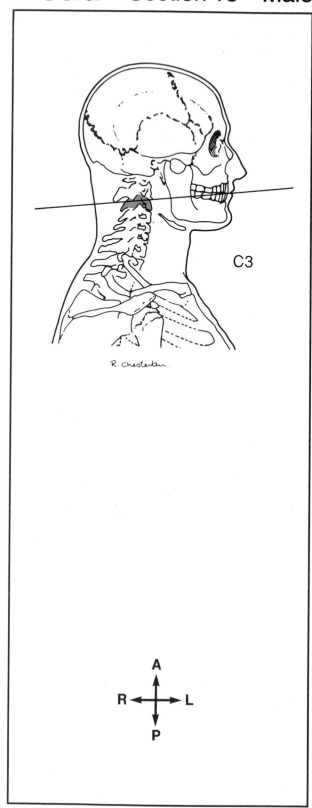

C3

R. Chesterton

A
R ←→ L
P

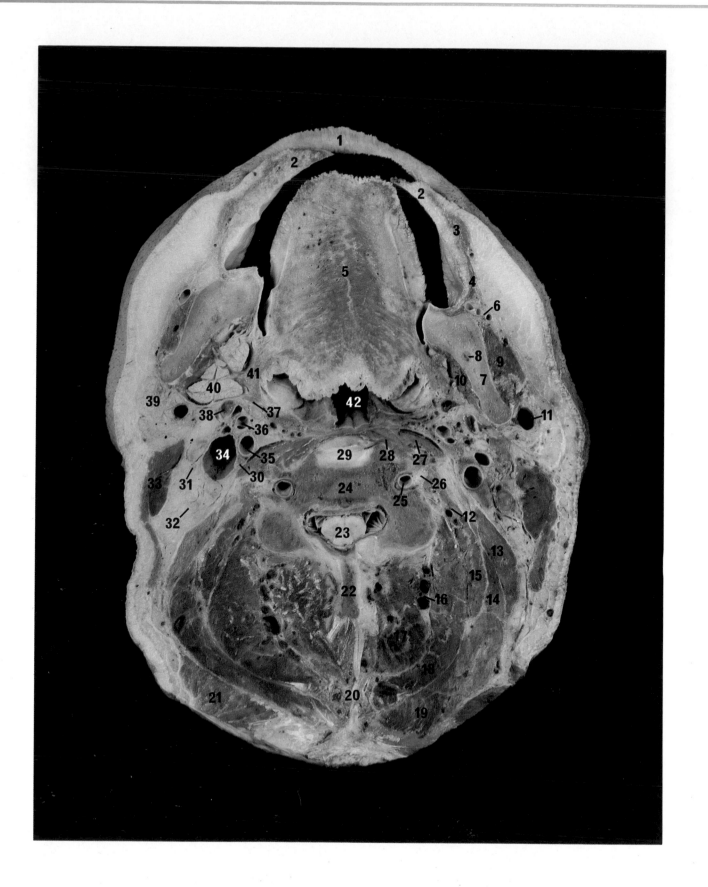

1 Upper lip
2 Lower lip
3 Orbicularis oris
4 Buccinator
5 Transverse intrinsic muscle of tongue
6 Facial artery and vein
7 Ramus of mandible
8 Inferior alveolar artery, vein and nerve (V^{III}) within mandibular canal
9 Masseter
10 Medial pterygoid
11 Retromandibular vein
12 Scalenus medius
13 Levator scapulae
14 Splenius cervicis
15 Longissimus capitis
16 Deep cervical vein
17 Semispinalis cervicis
18 Semispinalis capitis
19 Splenius capitis
20 Ligamentum nuchae
21 Trapezius
22 Spine of third cervical vertebra
23 Spinal cord within dural sheath
24 Body of third cervical vertebra
25 Vertebral artery and vein within foramen transversarium

26 Anterior primary ramus of third cervical nerve
27 Longus capitis
28 Longus colli
29 Part of intervertebral disc between second and third cervical vertebrae
30 Vagus nerve (X)
31 Accessory nerve (XI)
32 Deep cervical lymph node
33 Sternocleidomastoid
34 Internal jugular vein
35 Internal carotid artery
36 External carotid artery
37 Stylohyoid
38 Tendon of digastric
39 Parotid gland
40 Submandibular salivary gland
41 Styloglossus entering tongue
42 Oropharynx

43 Genioglossus
44 Constrictor muscle of pharynx
45 Base of tongue
46 Mylohyoid
47 Hyoglossus
48 External jugular vein

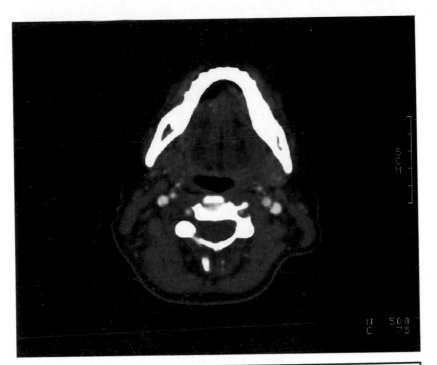

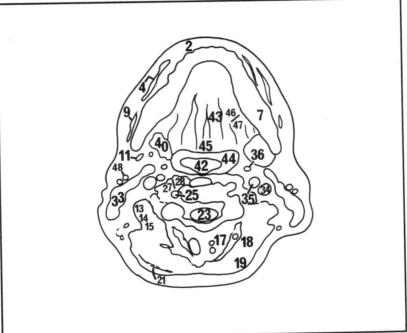

NOTES

This section passes between the lips (1, 2), the body of the third cervical vertebra (24) and its spine (22). The CT image is from a different subject and comes from the series which traverse the neck. This is because few cranial CT runs extend as caudal as this level. Moreover, artefacts from the amalgam of dental fillings often obscure this region. In the CT image, bolus enhancement with intravenous iodinated contrast medium has opacified the major vessels (34–36) and assists in their identification.

The submandibular salivary gland (40) lies against the ramus of the mandible (7) at its angle, separated by the medial pterygoid muscle (10). Its close relationship to the parotid gland (39) is well demonstrated; it is separated from the latter only by the fascial sheet of the sphenomandibular ligament.

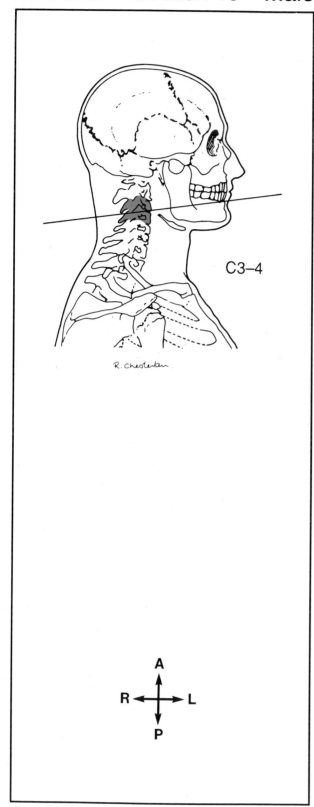

C3–4

R. Chesterton

A
R ← → L
P

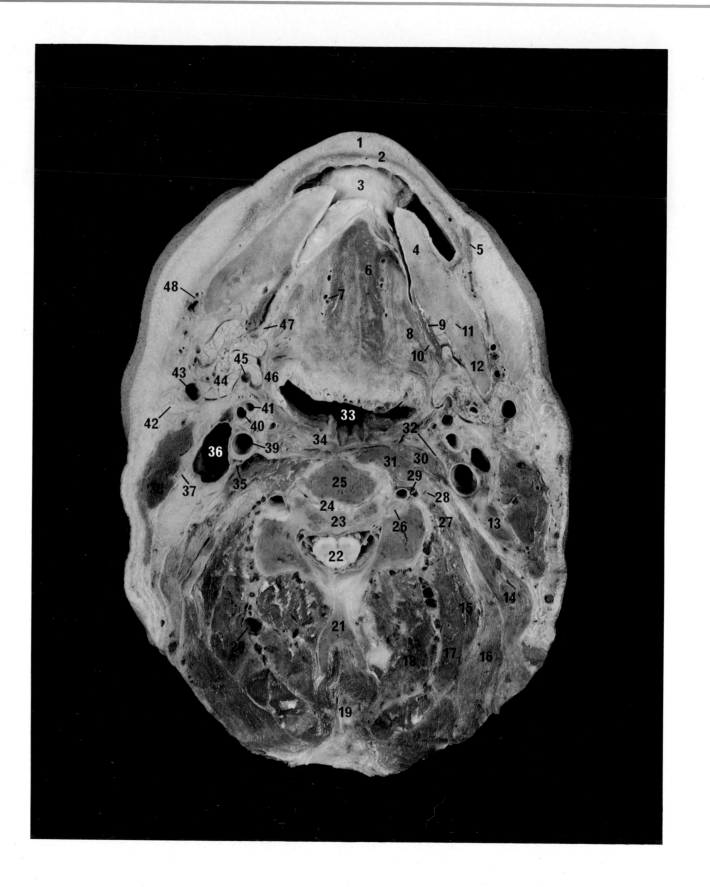

1 Lower lip
2 Orbicularis oris
3 Under surface of tongue
4 Body of mandible
5 Depressor anguli oris
6 Genioglossus
7 Lingual artery and vein
8 Hyoglossus
9 Mylohyoid
10 Lingual nerve (V^{III})
11 Inferior alveolar nerve (V^{III}) within mandibular canal
12 Ramus of mandible
13 Cervical lymph nodes
14 Levator scapulae
15 Splenius cervicis
16 Splenius capitis
17 Semispinalis capitis
18 Semispinalis cervicis
19 Ligamentum nuchae
20 Deep cervical vein
21 Spine of fourth cervical vertebra
22 Spinal cord within dural sheath
23 Part of body of fourth cervical vertebra
24 Part of intervertebral disc between third and fourth cervical vertebrae
25 Part of body of third cervical vertebra
26 Dorsal root ganglion of fourth cervical nerve

27 Scalenus medius
28 Scalenus anterior origin
29 Vertebral artery and vein within foramen transversarium
30 Longus capitis
31 Longus colli
32 Prevertebral fascia
33 Oropharynx
34 Constrictor muscles of pharynx
35 Vagus nerve (X)
36 Internal jugular vein
37 Accessory nerve (XI)
38 Sternocleidomastoid
39 Internal carotid artery
40 External carotid artery
41 Origin of facial artery
42 Parotid gland
43 Retromandibular vein
44 Submandibular salivary gland – superficial lobe
45 Tendon of digastric
46 Styloglossus
47 Deep lobe of submandibular salivary gland
48 Facial artery and vein

49 Platysma
50 Hyoid bone
51 External jugular vein

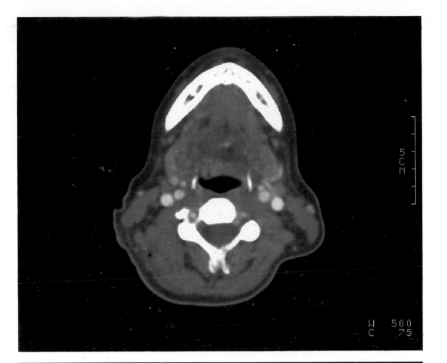

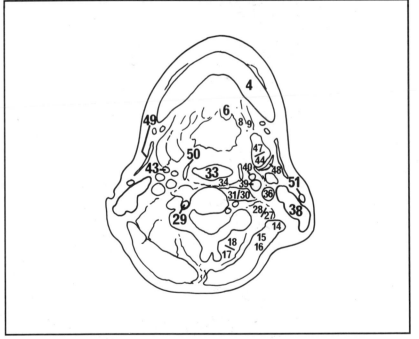

NOTES

This section passes through the upper border of the lower lip (1), genioglossus at the base of the tongue (6) and the cartilagenous disc between the third and fourth cervical vertebrae (24).

The prevertebral fascia (32) invests the front of the bodies of the cervical vertebrae, the prevertebral muscles (30, 31) and the scalene muscles (27, 28). It forms an almost avascular transverse plane behind the pharynx (33) and the great vessels (36, 39).

The facial artery at its origin from the external carotid artery (40) is seen at (41). It arches over the submandibular salivary gland (44) to cross the lower border of the mandible (4) where its pulse is palpable (48).

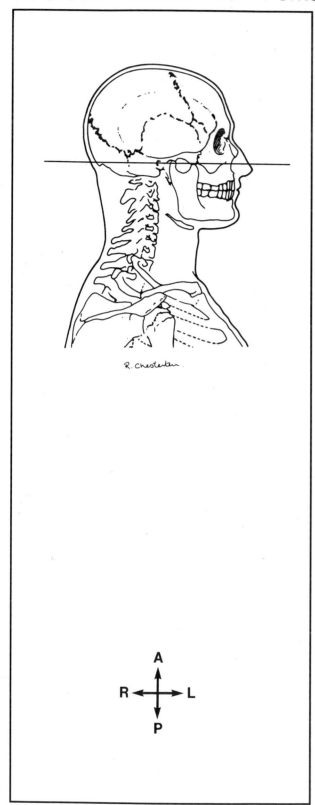

R. Chesterton

A
R ← → L
P

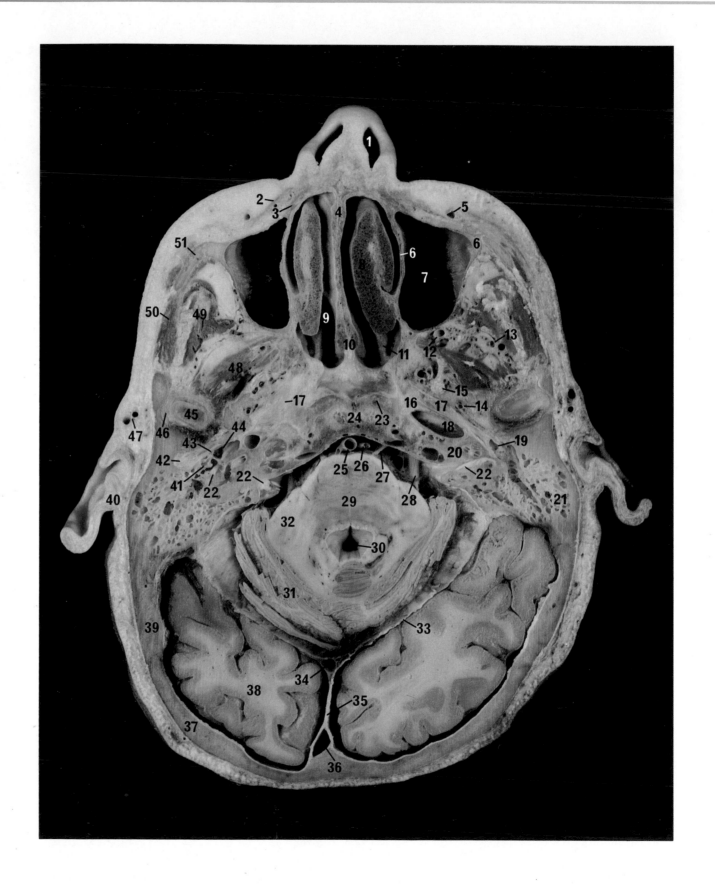

1 Vestibule of nose
2 Levator labii superioris alaeque nasi
3 Levator labii superioris
4 Cartilage of nasal septum
5 Facial vein
6 Maxilla
7 Maxillary sinus (antrum of Highmore)
8 Inferior nasal concha
9 Middle meatus
10 Vomer
11 Middle nasal concha
12 Maxillary artery
13 Pterygoid branch of maxillary artery
14 Middle meningeal artery
15 Mandibular nerve (V^{III})
16 Greater wing of sphenoid
17 Cartilaginous roof of auditory (eustachian) tube
18 Internal carotid artery
19 Junction of auditory tube and tympanic cavity
20 Petrous temporal bone
21 Mastoid air cells
22 Facial nerve (VII)
23 Longus capitis
24 Body of sphenoid
25 Basilar artery
26 Anterior inferior cerebellar artery
27 Abducent nerve (VI)
28 Trigeminal nerve (V)
29 Pons cerebri

30 Fourth ventricle
31 Cerebellum
32 Middle cerebellar peduncle
33 Tentorium cerebelli
34 Straight sinus
35 Falx cerebri
36 Superior sagittal sinus
37 Occipital bone (squamous part)
38 Occipital lobe of cerebrum
39 Squamous part of temporal bone
40 Pinna of ear
41 Malleus and incus
42 External auditory meatus
43 Tympanic membrane
44 Cavity of middle ear
45 Head of mandible
46 Temporomandibular joint
47 Superficial temporal artery and vein
48 Lateral pterygoid
49 Temporalis and tendon
50 Masseter
51 Zygomatic process of maxilla

52 Internal jugular vein (at origin)
53 Occipital bone (basilar part)
54 Postnasal space
55 Coronoid process of mandible

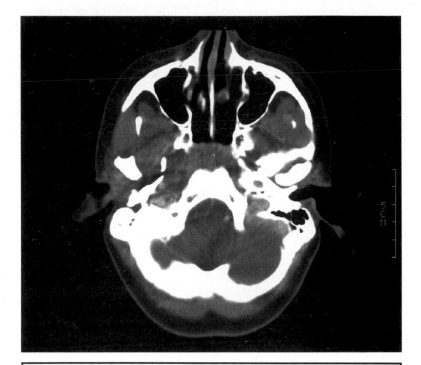

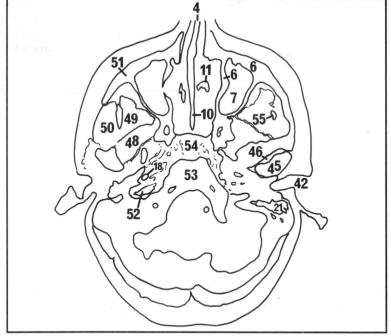

NOTES

This section passes through the vestibule of the nose (1), the inferior nasal concha (8), the temporomandibular joint (46), the pons (29) and the occipital lobe of the cerebrum (38).

This CT image is the most cranial of a series designed principally to demonstrate the great vessels of the neck. The angulation of the CT series does not tally exactly with the sections; some of the anatomical features of the neck are therefore better seen on the cranial CT image series.

The maxillary sinus (the antrum of Highmore) within the maxilla (7) is well demonstrated. Its orifice lies at a higher plane and drains into the middle meatus (9) below the bulla ethmoidalis. The fact that the opening of this antrum is situated at this high level accounts for the poor drainage and consequent frequency of infection.

Note that the lateral pterygoid muscle (48) inserts not only into a depression on the front of the neck of the mandible, but also into the articular capsule of the temporomandibular joint (46) and also its articular disc.

The postnasal space (54) lies between the nasopharynx and the basi-occiput (53) together with the anterior arch of the atlas. As well as containing the prevertebral muscles, this space also contains variable quantities of lymphoid tissue (the pharyngeal tonsil, or adenoids). The size of the space is readily assessed on a lateral radiograph of the region. It is usually very narrow in adults (see section 23), but can be very prominent in young children whose adenoids are often very large.

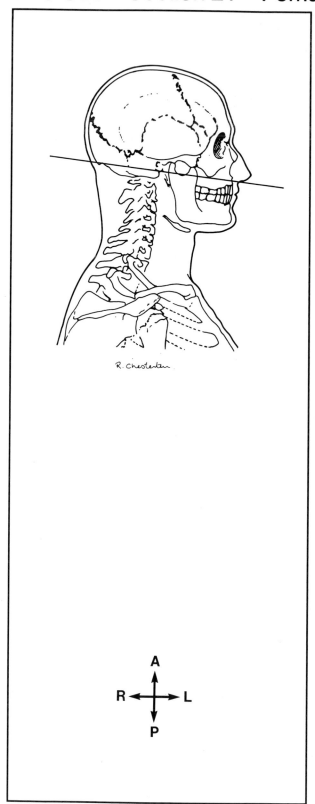

R. Chesterton.

A
R ← → L
P

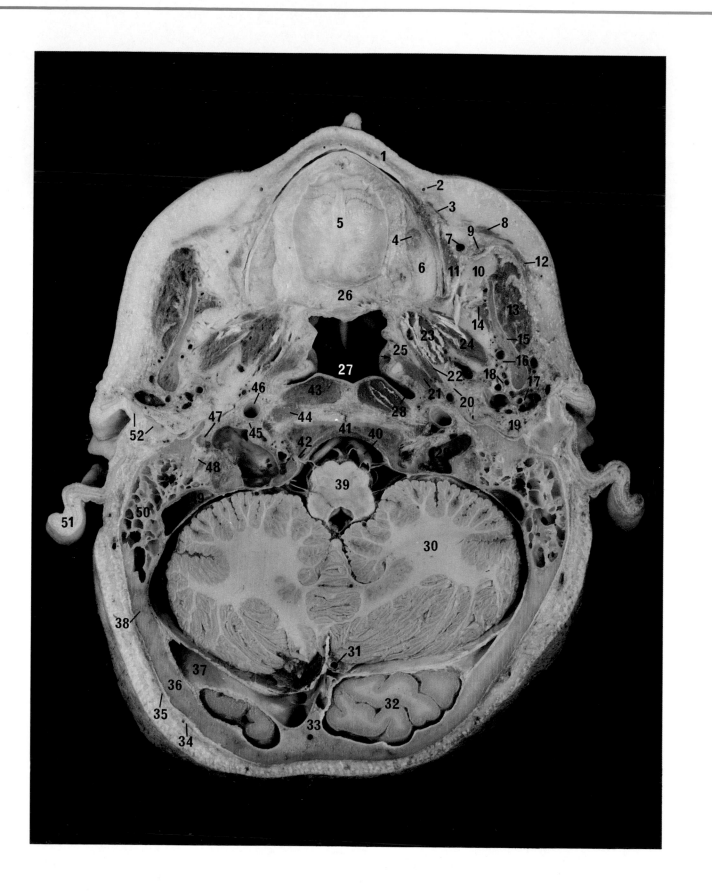

1 Orbicularis oris
2 Facial artery
3 Levator labii superioris
4 Mucosa of maxillary antrum
5 Hard palate
6 Alveolar process of maxilla
7 Facial vein
8 Zygomaticus major
9 Parotid duct
10 Buccal fat pad
11 Buccinator
12 Accessory parotid gland
13 Masseter
14 Temporalis and tendon
15 Ramus of mandible
16 Inferior alveolar artery and vein
17 Superficial temporal artery and vein
18 Maxillary artery and vein
19 Parotid gland
20 Lingual nerve, inferior alveolar nerve and nerve to mylohyoid (V^{III})
21 Levator veli palatini
22 Tensor veli palatini
23 Medial pterygoid
24 Lateral pterygoid
25 Orifice of auditory tube (eustachian tube) arrowed
26 Soft palate
27 Nasopharynx
28 Pharyngeal recess (fossa of Rosenmueller)
29 Internal jugular vein at origin
30 Cerebellum

31 Straight sinus at junction of tentorium cerebelli, falx cerebri and falx cerebelli
32 Occipital lobe of cerebrum
33 Internal occipital crest
34 Occipital artery and vein
35 Occipitofrontalis
36 Squamous part of occipital bone
37 Transverse sinus
38 Occipitomastoid suture
39 Medulla oblongata
40 Vertebral artery
41 Clivus of the basilar part of the occipital bone
42 Hypoglossal nerve (XII)
43 Longus capitis
44 Rectus capitis anterior
45 Glossopharyngeal nerve (IX), vagus nerve (X) and accessory nerve (XI)
46 Internal carotid artery
47 Styloid process
48 Facial nerve (VII)
49 Sigmoid sinus
50 Mastoid air cells of the temporal bone
51 Pinna of ear
52 Cartilage of external auditory meatus

53 Dens (odontoid process) of axis (second cervical vertebra)
54 Sternocleidomastoid
55 Semispinalis capitis
56 Splenius capitis
57 Mastoid process

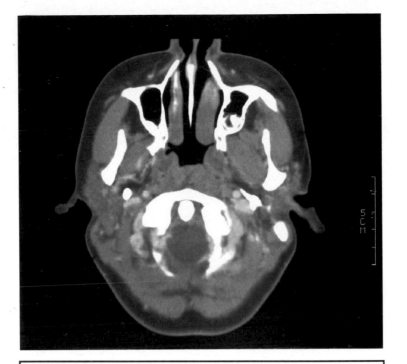

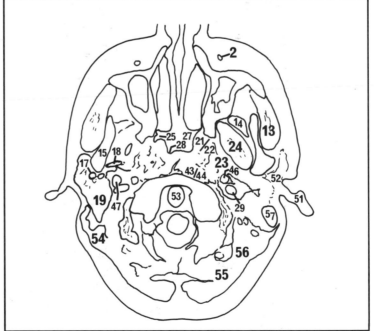

NOTES

This section passes through the alveolar process of the maxilla (6) to reveal the hard palate (5) in its entirety. It then traverses the upper part of the ramus of the mandible (15), the mastoid air cells (50), the medulla oblongata (39), cerebellum (30) and the posterior tip of the occipital lobe (32).

The floor of the maxillary sinus is formed by the alveolar process of the maxilla; several conical elevations, corresponding to the roots of the first and second molar teeth, project into the floor. An example of this is demonstrated here (4). Indeed, the floor is sometimes perforated by one or more of these molar roots.

This section gives a good view of the parotid duct (9) as it arches medially to penetrate the buccinator (11) and to enter the mouth at the level of the second upper molar tooth. The parotid duct is accompanied by a small, more or less detached, part of the gland which lies above the duct as it crosses the masseter; this is named the accessory part of the gland (12).

This section passes through the junctional zone between the falx cerebri, separating the occipital lobes of the brain (32), the falx cerebelli, separating the lobes of the cerebellum (30) and the tentorium cerebelli, which roofs the cerebellum. The straight sinus (31) is seen in section as it lies in the line of junction of the falx cerebri and tentorium cerebelli. The transverse sinus (37) lies in the attached margin of the tentorium cerebelli.

The facial nerve (within the stylomastoid foramen) is well demonstrated (48) in its immediate lateral relationship to the root of the styloid process (47).

Note that the orifice of the auditory tube (25) lies anterior to a depression – the pharyngeal recess (28). This helps to keep the orifice of the tube clear of secretions in the supine position.

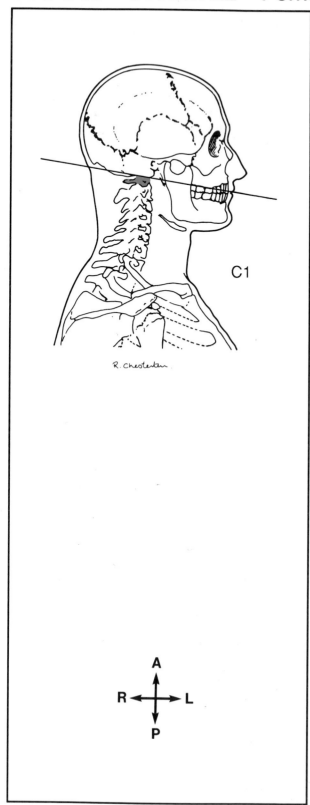

C1

R. Chesterton

A
R ← → L
P

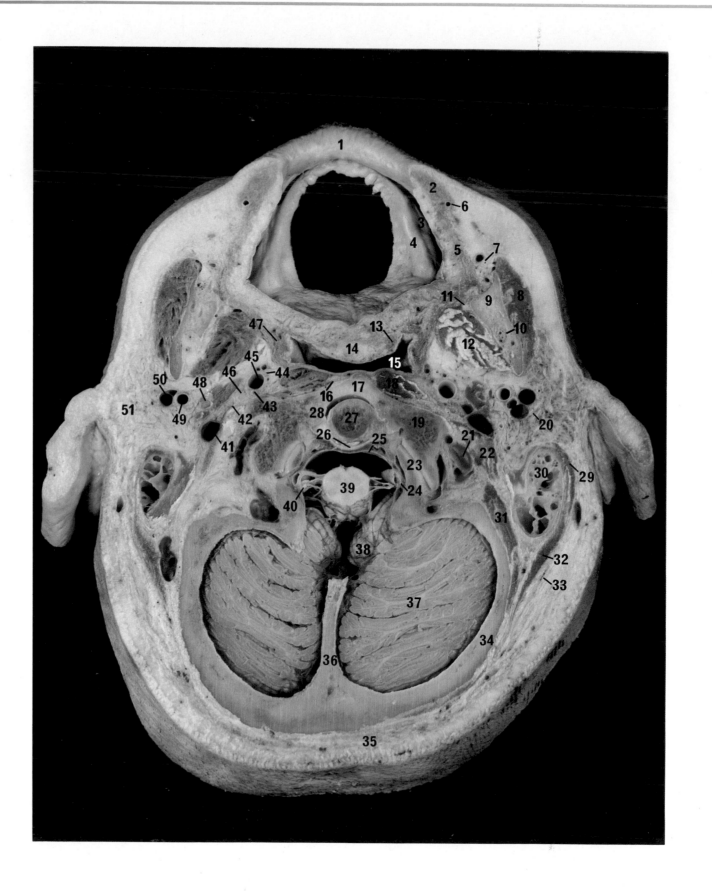

1 Upper lip
2 Orbicularis oris
3 Vestibule of mouth
4 Alveolus
5 Buccinator
6 Superior labial artery
7 Facial artery and vein
8 Masseter
9 Ramus of mandible
10 Inferior alveolar artery, vein and nerve (V^{III}) within mandibular canal
11 Lingual nerve (V^{III})
12 Medial pterygoid
13 Tensor veli palatini
14 Soft palate
15 Nasopharynx
16 Anterior atlanto-occipital membrane
17 Anterior arch of atlas (first cervical vertebra)
18 Longus capitis
19 Lateral mass of atlas (first cervical vertebra)
20 Facial nerve (VII)
21 Roof of third part of vertebral artery
22 Rectus capitis lateralis
23 Atlanto-occipital joint
24 fourth part of vertebral artery
25 Membrana tectoria
26 Superior longitudinal band of cruciform ligament
27 Dens of axis (odontoid process) (second cervical vertebra)

28 Atlanto-axial joint
29 Sternocleidomastoid
30 Mastoid air cells of temporal bone
31 Posterior belly of digastric
32 Longissimus capitis
33 Splenius capitis
34 Squamous part of occipital bone
35 Trapezius
36 Internal occipital crest of occipital bone
37 Hemisphere of cerebellum
38 Tonsil of cerebellum
39 Spinal cord
40 Spinal root of accessory nerve
41 Internal jugular vein
42 Accessory nerve (XI) and hypoglossal nerve (XII)
43 Vagus nerve (X)
44 Sympathetic chain
45 Internal carotid artery
46 Glossopharyngeal nerve (IX)
47 Superior constrictor muscle of pharynx
48 Styloid process
49 External carotid artery
50 Retromandibular vein at bifurcation
51 Parotid gland

52 Semispinalis capitis
53 Parapharyngeal space

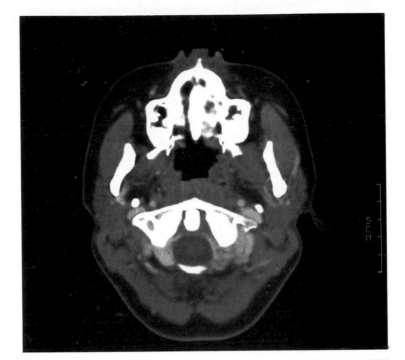

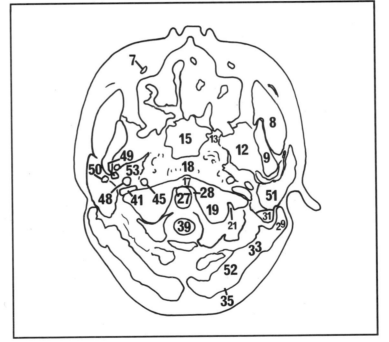

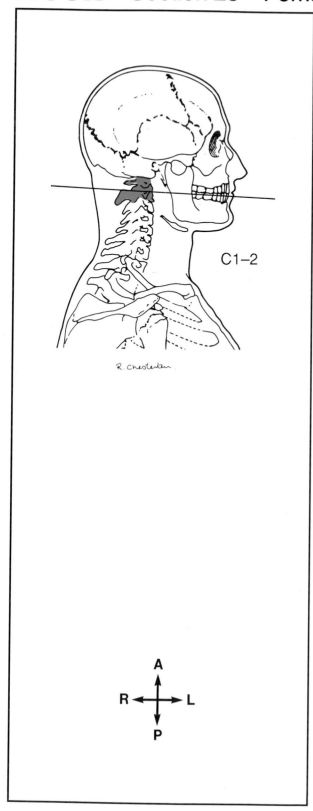

C1–2

R. Chesterton

A
R ← → L
P

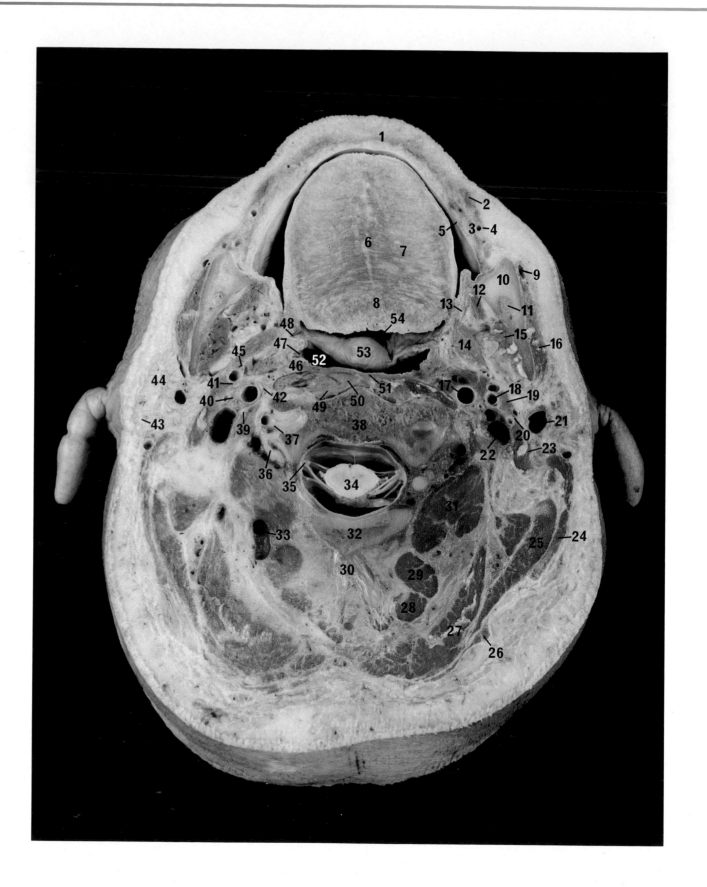

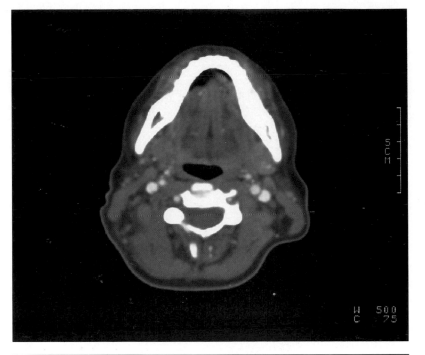

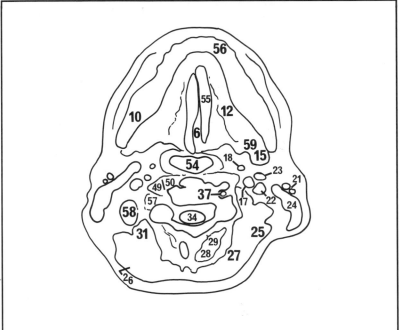

NOTES

This section passes through the tongue (6) and the body of the axis, the second cervical vertebra (38).

This section gives a useful appreciation of the inferior alveolar nerve and its accompanying vessels within the mandibular canal (11). Note also the vertebral artery in its second part, together with its accompanying vein, within the foramen transversarium (37). The further course of this artery, in its third and fourth part, can be seen in section 22.

Note how close the posterior wall of the nasopharynx (52) lies to the body of the axis (38) – and also to the anterior arch of the atlas in the previous section. The prevertebral space is thus normally very narrow on a lateral radiograph of the adult cervical spine (see section 20).

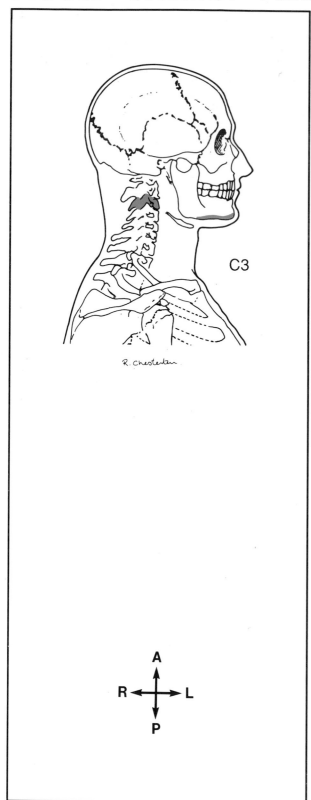

C3

R. Chesterton

A
R ← → L
P

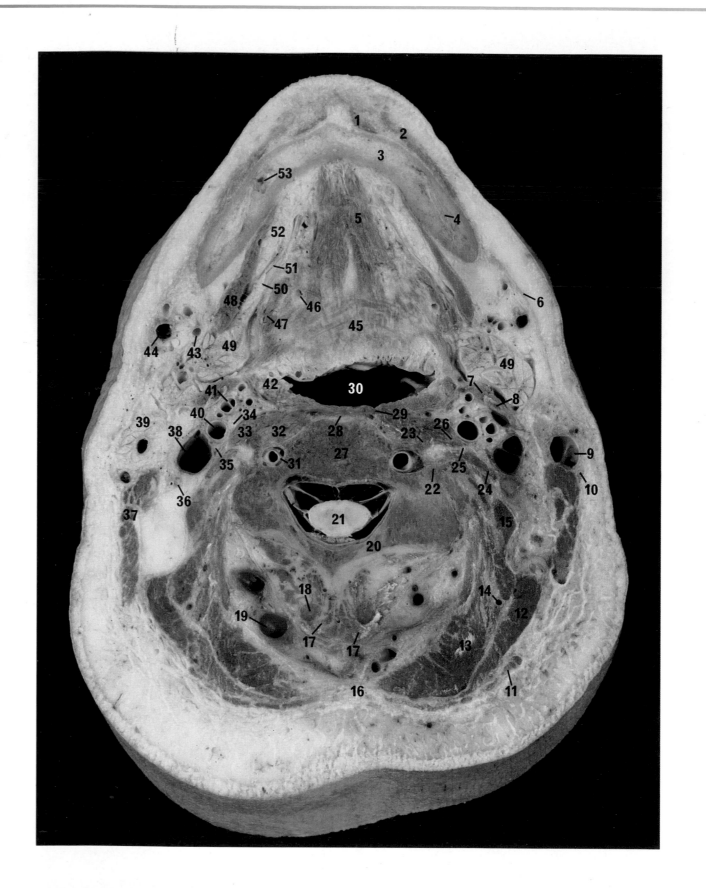

1 Mentalis
2 Orbicularis oris
3 Mandible
4 Inferior alveolar nerve (V^{III})
5 Genioglossus
6 Platysma
7 Posterior belly of digastric
8 Stylohyoid ligament
9 External jugular vein
10 Great auricular nerve
11 Trapezius
12 Splenius
13 Semispinalis capitis
14 Occipital artery
15 Levator scapulae
16 Ligamentum nuchae
17 Bifid spine of third cervical vertebra
18 Semispinalis cervicis
19 Occipital vein
20 Lamina of third cervical vertebra
21 Spinal cord within dural sheath
22 Posterior tubercle of transverse process of third cervical vertebra
23 Anterior tubercle of transverse process of third cervical vertebra
24 Scalenus medius
25 Anterior primary ramus of third cervical nerve
26 Scalenus anterior
27 Body of third cervical vertebra

28 Anterior longitudinal ligament
29 Superior constrictor muscle of pharynx
30 Oropharynx
31 Vertebral artery and vein within foramen transversarium
32 Longus colli
33 Longus capitis
34 Vagus nerve (X)
35 Sympathetic chain
36 Accessory nerve (XI)
37 Sternocleidomastoid
38 Internal jugular vein
39 Parotid gland
40 Internal carotid artery
41 External carotid artery
42 Palatine tonsil
43 Facial artery
44 Facial vein
45 Intrinsic transverse muscle of tongue
46 Lingual artery
47 Hyoglossus
48 Mylohyoid
49 Submandibular gland
50 Lingual nerve (V^{III})
51 Submandibular duct
52 Sublingual gland
53 Inferior alveolar artery, vein and nerve within mandibular canal

54 Hyoid

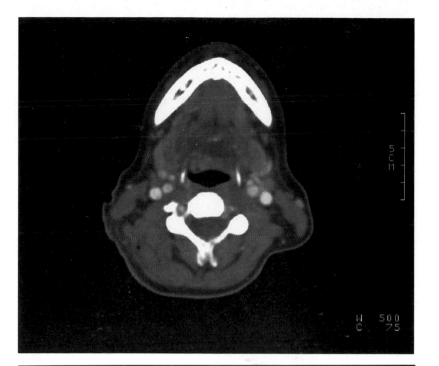

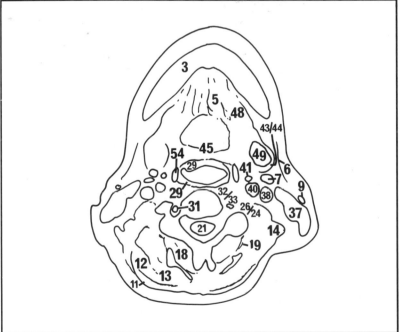

NOTES

This section passes through the lower border of the body of the mandible (3) the oropharynx (30) and the third cervical vertebra (27).

It demonstrates how the parotid gland (39) projects deeply towards the side wall of the oropharynx (30). Indeed, a tumour of the deep portion of the gland may project into the tonsillar fossa and displace the palatine tonsil (42) medially.

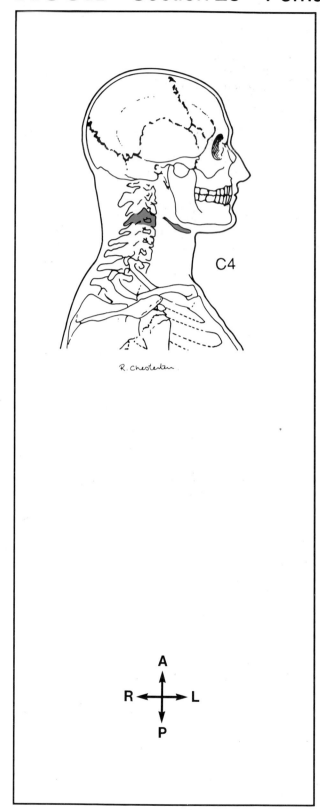

C4

R. Chesterton

A
R ←→ L
P

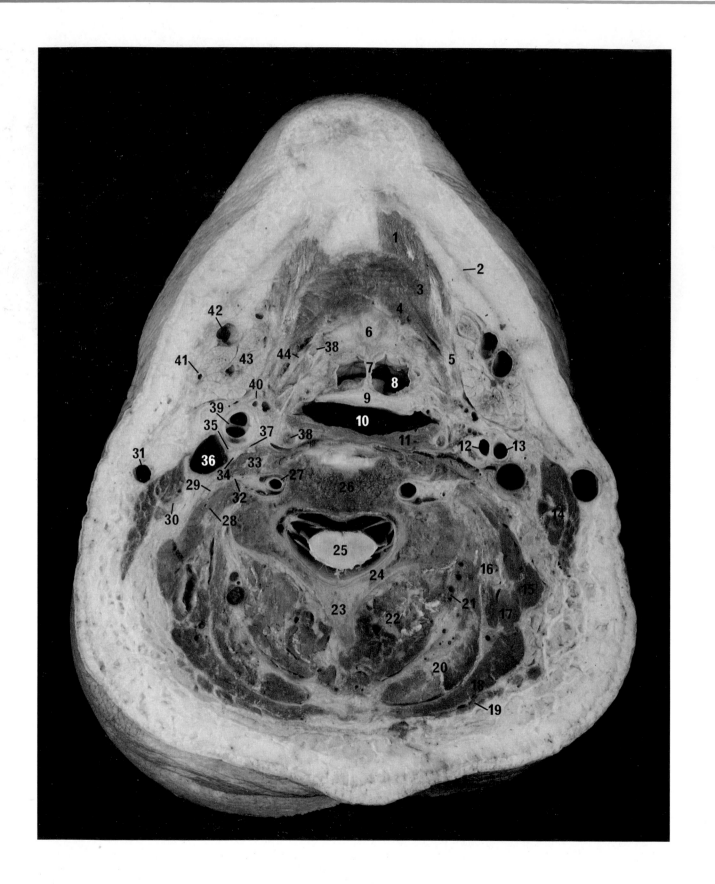

1 Anterior belly of digastric	27 Vertebral artery and vein within foramen transversarium
2 Platysma	28 Scalenus medius
3 Mylohyoid	29 Anterior primary ramus of third cervical nerve
4 Hyoglossus	
5 Tendon of digastric	30 Accessory nerve (XI)
6 Base of tongue	31 External jugular vein
7 Glosso-epiglottic fold	32 Anterior primary ramus of fourth cervical nerve
8 Vallecula	
9 Epiglottis	33 Scalenus anterior
10 Laryngopharynx	34 Phrenic nerve
11 Middle constrictor muscle of pharynx	35 Vagus nerve (X)
	36 Internal jugular vein
12 Left external carotid artery	37 Sympathetic chain
13 Left internal carotid artery	38 Hyoid
14 Sternocleidomastoid	39 Right common carotid artery at bifurcation
15 Levator scapulae	
16 Longissimus capitis and cervicis	40 Superior thyroid artery
	41 Facial artery
17 Splenius cervicis	42 Facial vein
18 Splenius capitis	43 Submandibular salivary gland
19 Trapezius	
20 Semispinalis capitis	44 Lingual artery
21 Deep cervical artery and vein	
	45 Mandible
22 Semispinalis cervicis	46 Common carotid artery
23 Spine of fourth cervical vertebra	47 Pre-epiglottic space
	48 Superior cornu of thyroid cartilage
24 Lamina of fourth cervical vertebra	
25 Spinal cord within dural sheath	49 Aryepiglottic fold
	50 Piriform fossa
26 Body of fourth cervical vertebra	

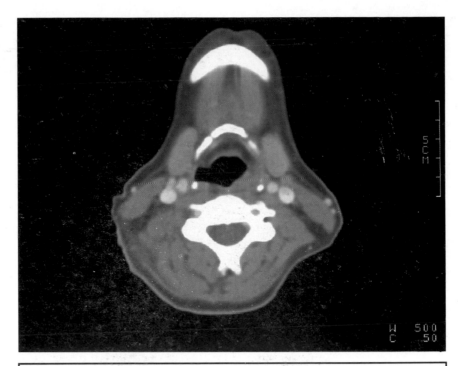

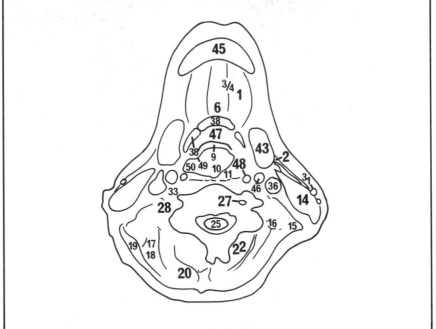

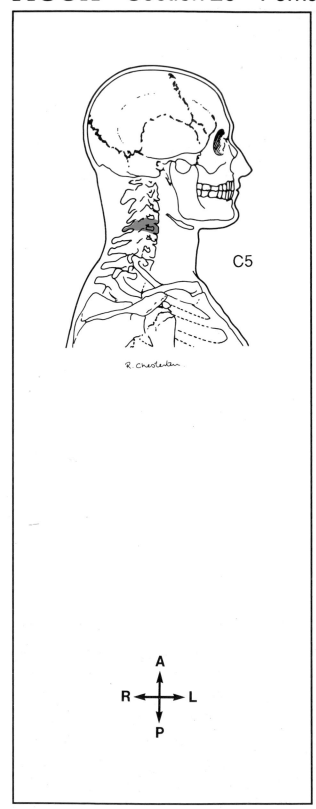

C5

R. Chesterton

A
R ← → L
P

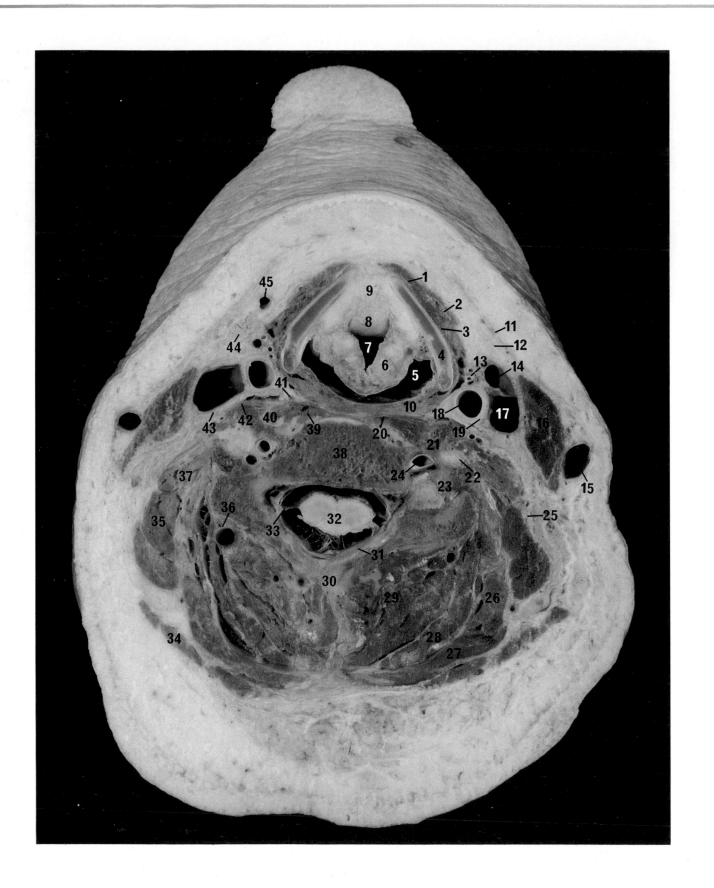

1 Sternohyoid
2 Omohyoid
3 Thyrohyoid
4 Lamina of thyroid cartilage
5 Laryngopharynx
6 Corniculate cartilage
7 Vestibule of larynx
8 Epiglottis
9 Pre-epiglottic space (fat-filled)
10 Inferior constrictor muscle of pharynx
11 Platysma
12 Investing fascia of neck
13 Superior thyroid artery and vein
14 Common facial vein
15 External jugular vein
16 Sternocleidomastoid
17 Internal jugular vein
18 Common carotid artery
19 Vagus nerve (X)
20 Prevertebral fascia
21 Anterior tubercle of fifth cervical vertebra
22 Ventral ramus of fifth cervical nerve
23 Posterior tubercle of fifth cervical vertebra
24 Vertebral artery and vein within foramen transversarium
25 Accessory nerve (XI)
26 Splenius cervicis

27 Splenius capitis
28 Semispinalis capitis
29 Erector spinae
30 Spine of fifth cervical vertebra
31 Lamina of fifth cervical vertebra
32 Spinal cord within dural sheath
33 Ligamentum denticulatum
34 Trapezius
35 Levator scapulae
36 Deep cervical artery and vein
37 Scalenus medius
38 Body of fifth cervical vertebra
39 Longus colli
40 Longus capitis
41 Sympathetic chain
42 Scalenus anterior
43 Phrenic nerve
44 Submandibular salivary gland
45 Anterior jugular vein

46 Inferior horn of thyroid cartilage
47 Arytenoid cartilage
48 Cricoid cartilage
49 Vocal fold
50 Anterior border of thyroid cartilage

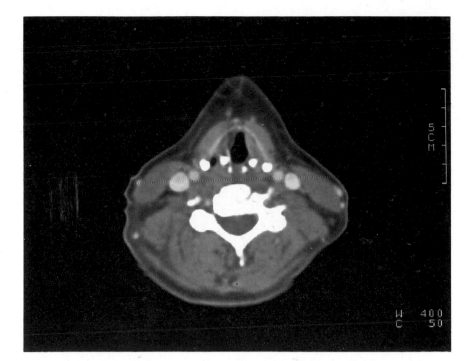

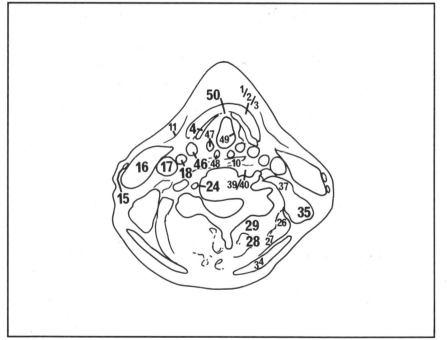

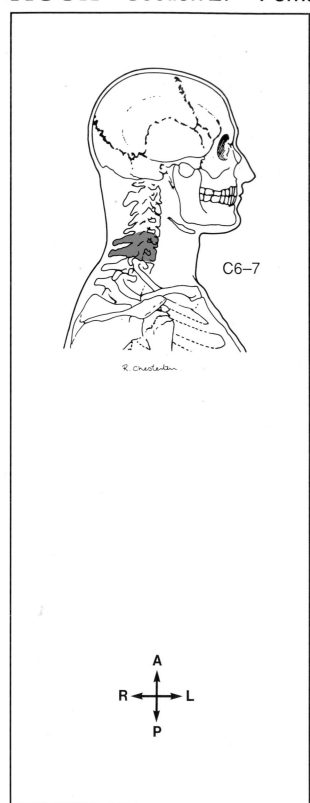

C6–7

R. Chesterton

A
R ← → L
P

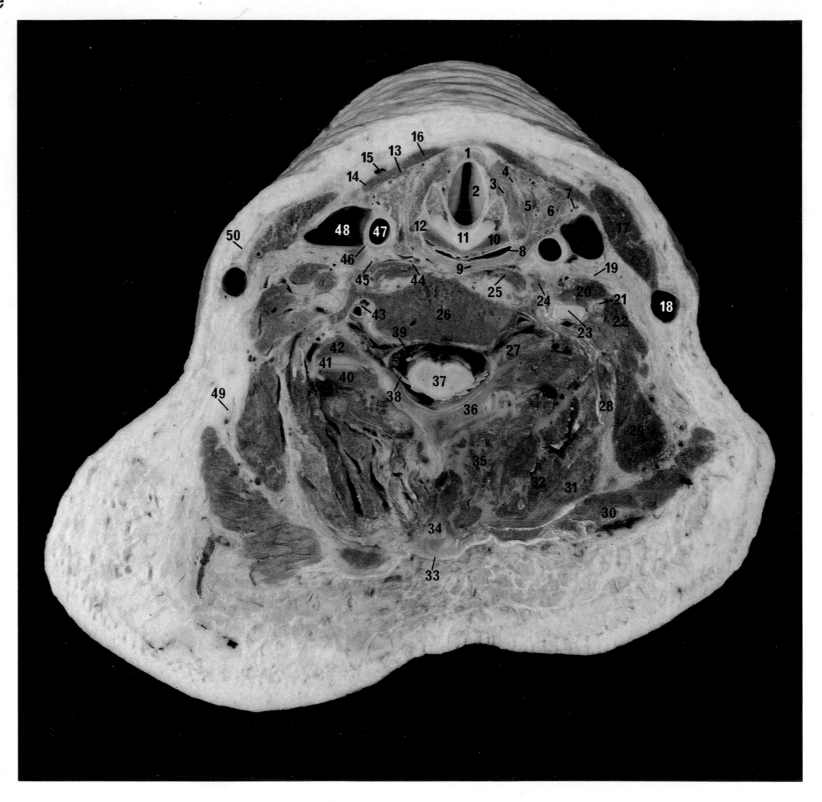

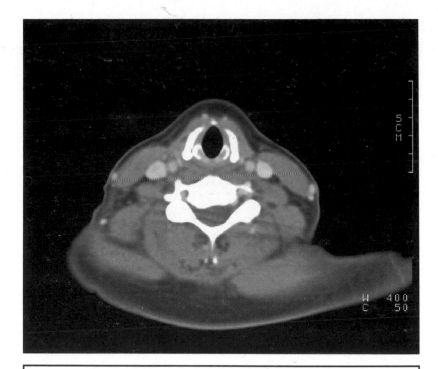

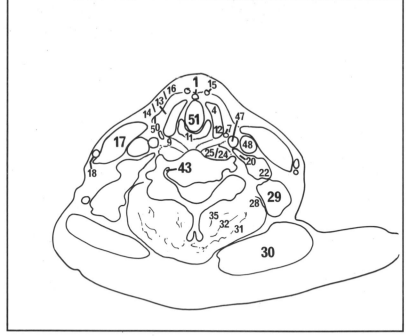

NOTES

This section passes through the body of the sixth cervical vertebra (26) and traverses the cricoid cartilage (11). The cricoid is the only complete ring of cartilage throughout the respiratory system, but the plane of this section is above the narrow arch of the cricoid and only passes through its posterior lamina.

This section, together with the following one, provides a good appreciation of the relationships of the lateral lobe of the thyroid gland (6). Here, it is seen to be overlapped superficially by the strap muscles – the sternohyoid (16), omohyoid (14) and, on a deeper plane, the sternothyroid (13). Medially, it lies against the larynx and laryngopharynx (8) and posteriorly it lies against the common carotid artery (47) and internal jugular vein (48). (See also CT image, section 28.)

Note the demonstration of the relationship of the phrenic nerve (19) to the anterior aspect of the scalenus anterior (20). The nerve is bound down to the underlying muscle by the overlying prevertebral fascia (44).

The ventral rami (21 and 23) of C5 and C6 together with C7, C8 and T1, form the brachial plexus; those of C1–4 form the cervical plexus.

The inferior surfaces of the vocal folds (2) can be seen within the larynx (see CT image, section 26). The vestibular folds (false cords), which lie cranial to the vestibule of the larynx, are situated more cranially to this section.

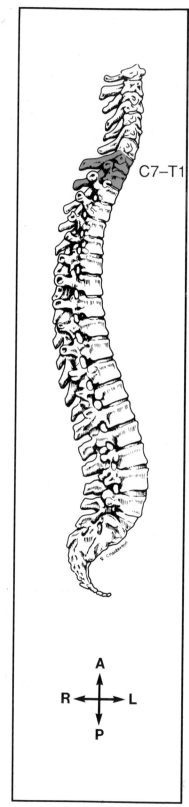

C7–T1

A
R ← → L
P

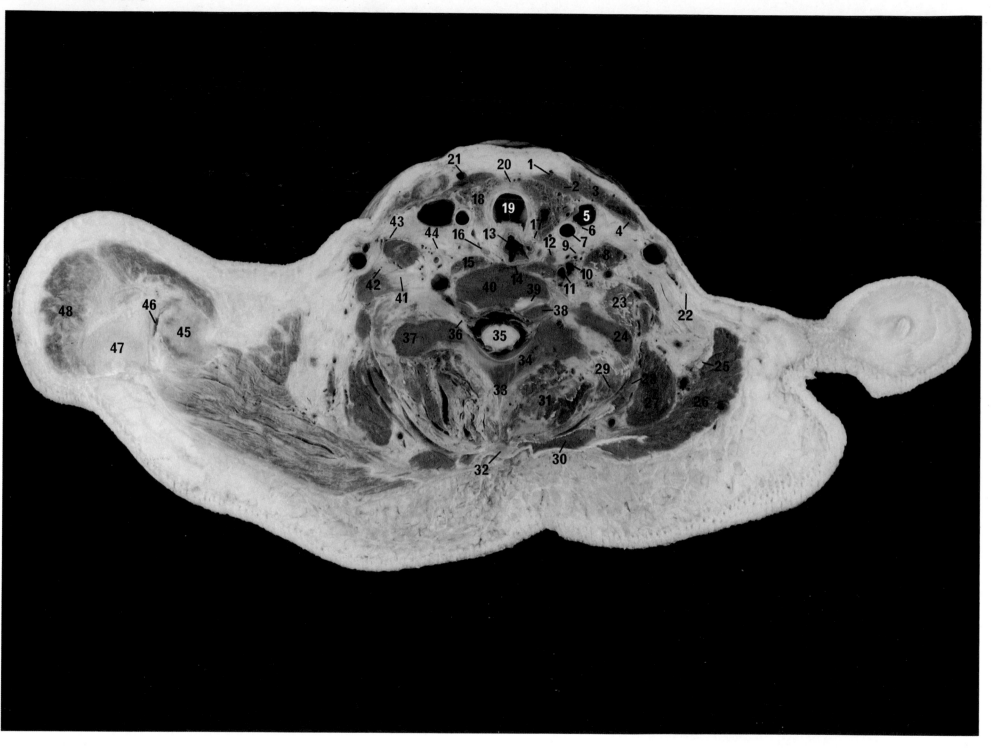

1 Sternohyoid
2 Sternothyroid
3 Sternocleidomastoid
4 Omohyoid
5 Internal jugular vein
6 Vagus nerve (X)
7 Common carotid artery
8 Scalenus anterior
9 Inferior thyroid artery
10 Vertebral vein
11 Vertebral artery
12 Deep cervical lymph node
13 Oesophagus
14 Prevertebral fascia
15 Longus colli
16 Parathyroid gland
17 Recurrent laryngeal nerve
18 Lateral lobe of thyroid gland
19 Trachea
20 Isthmus of thyroid gland
21 Anterior jugular vein
22 Investing (deep) fascia of the neck
23 Scalenus medius and posterior
24 Left first rib
25 Accessory nerve (XI)
26 Trapezius
27 Levator scapulae
28 Splenius
29 Semispinalis

30 Rhomboideus minor
31 Erector spinae
32 Ligamentum nuchae
33 Spinous process of first thoracic vertebra
34 Lamina of first thoracic vertebra
35 Spinal cord within dural sheath
36 Dorsal root ganglion of eighth cervical nerve
37 Transverse process of first thoracic vertebra
38 Part of body of first thoracic vertebra
39 Uncovertebral synovial joint between lip of T1 body and inferior aspect of C7
40 Body of seventh cervical vertebra
41 Ventral ramus of seventh cervical nerve
42 Ventral ramus of sixth cervical nerve
43 Phrenic nerve
44 Cervical sympathetic chain
45 Clavicle
46 Acromioclavicular joint
47 Acromion
48 Deltoid

49 External jugular vein

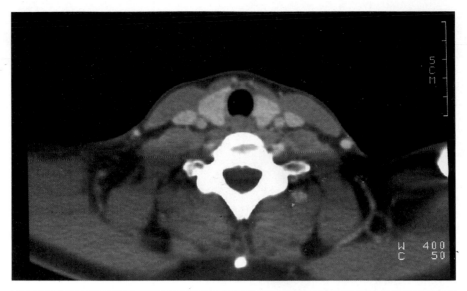

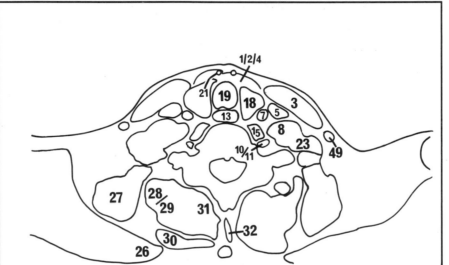

NOTES

This section passes through the body of the seventh cervical vertebra (40) and through the tip of the shoulder, so that a sliver of the clavicle (45) and adjacent acromioclavicular joint (46) are shown.

Taken in conjunction with the previous section, the relationships of the lateral lobe of the thyroid gland (18) are demonstrated. In this section, it is overlapped by the strap muscles (1, 2, 4) and by the sternocleidomastoid (3). Medially it lies against the trachea (19) and oesophagus (13), while posteriorly it rests against the common carotid artery (7) and internal jugular vein (5). The inferior thyroid artery (9) passes transversely behind the common carotid artery to reach the thyroid gland. Note also the important posterior relationship of the lobe of the thyroid gland to the recurrent laryngeal nerve (17), lying in the tracheo-oesophageal groove.

The parathyroid glands (16) are usually four in number but vary from two to six. The superior glands are fairly constant in position, at the middle of the posterior border of the thyroid lobe above the level at which the inferior thyroid artery crosses the recurrent laryngeal nerve. The inferior glands are most usually situated near the lower pole of the thyroid gland distal to the inferior thyroid artery, but aberrant glands may be found in front of the trachea, behind the oesophagus, buried in the thyroid gland or descended into the superior mediastinum in company with thymic tissue.

On the CT image the vertebral artery (11) is seen as it passes towards the gap between the foramina transversarium of the sixth and seventh cervical vertebrae.

The bodies of the cervical vertebrae and the superior aspect of T1 have raised lips (uncinate processes) on each lateral margin of their superior surfaces. These processes enclose the intervertebral disc and articulate (39) with the inferior aspect of the adjacent vertebral body; they are prone to degenerative disease which can lead to neurological problems.

71

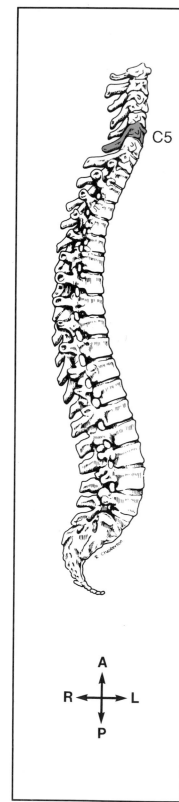

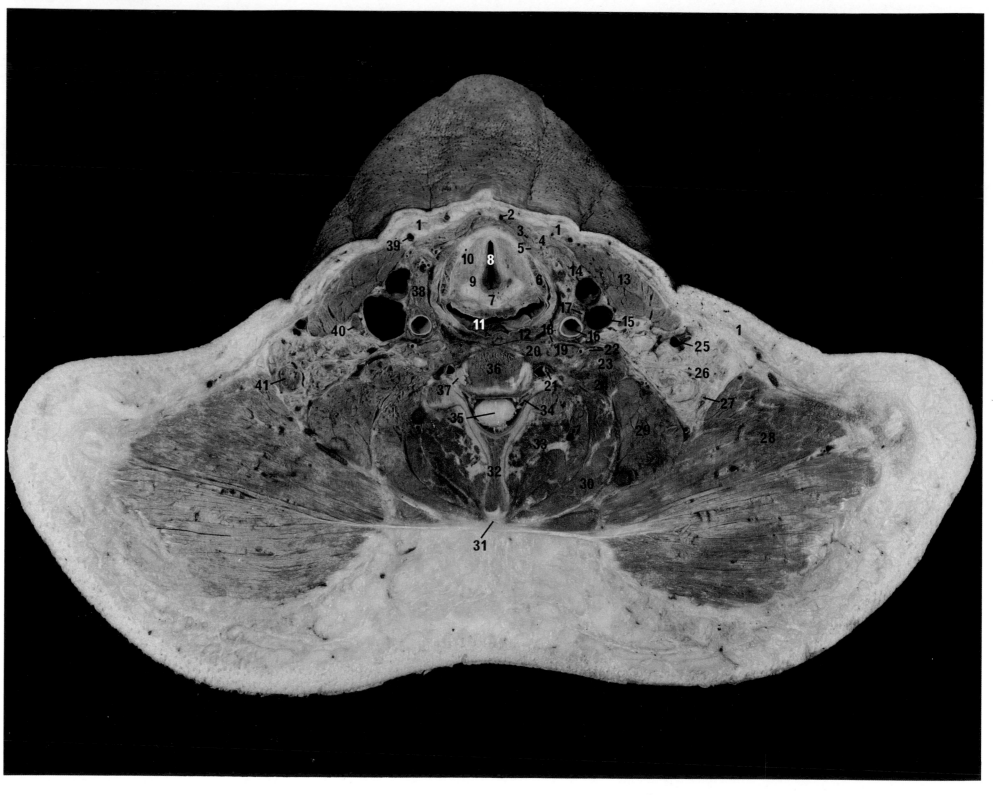

1 Platysma
2 Anterior jugular vein
3 Sternohyoid
4 Omohyoid
5 Sternothyroid
6 Thyroid cartilage
7 Cricoid cartilage
8 Rima glottidis
9 Arytenoid cartilage
10 Thyro-arytenoid
11 Pharynx
12 Inferior constrictor muscle of pharynx
13 Sternocleidomastoid
14 Common facial vein
15 Internal jugular vein
16 Common carotid artery
17 Vagus nerve (X)
18 Sympathetic chain
19 Longus capitis
20 Longus colli
21 Vertebral artery and vein within foramen transversarium
22 Phrenic nerve
23 Scalenus anterior
24 Scalenus medius and posterior
25 External jugular vein
26 Fat within posterior triangle
27 Accessory nerve (XI)
28 Trapezius
29 Levator scapulae
30 Splenius
31 Ligamentum nuchae
32 Spine of fifth cervical vertebra
33 Erector spinae
34 Root of sixth cervical nerve
35 Spinal cord within dural sheath
36 Body of fifth cervical vertebra
37 Neurocentral or uncovertebral synovial joint (of Lushka)
38 Lateral lobe of thyroid gland
39 Accessory anterior jugular vein
40 Lymph node of internal jugular chain
41 Cervical lymph node

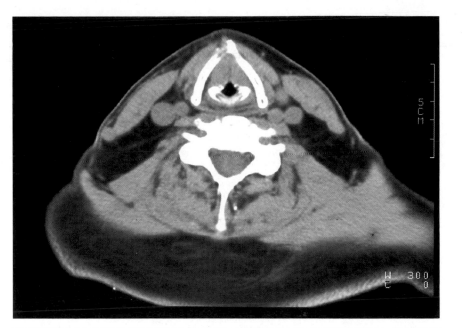

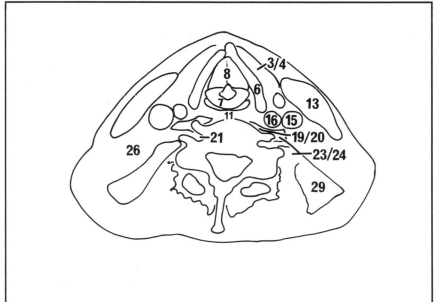

NOTES

This section passes through the body of the fifth cervical vertebra (36), immediately above the level of the shoulder joint. Here the fibres of the trapezius muscle (28) arch over the posterior extremity of the posterior triangle. Just below this level, at C6, lies the junction between the pharynx (11) and oesophagus, and the larynx (6,7,9) and the trachea. In both the section and CT image the pharynx (11) has a narrow anteroposterior diameter; it distends considerably during deglutition. On the CT image, the vocal cords of the rima glottidis (8) are adducted.

Not unusually, as in this case, the external jugular vein (39) is double.

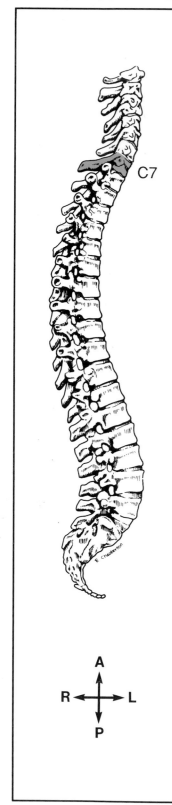

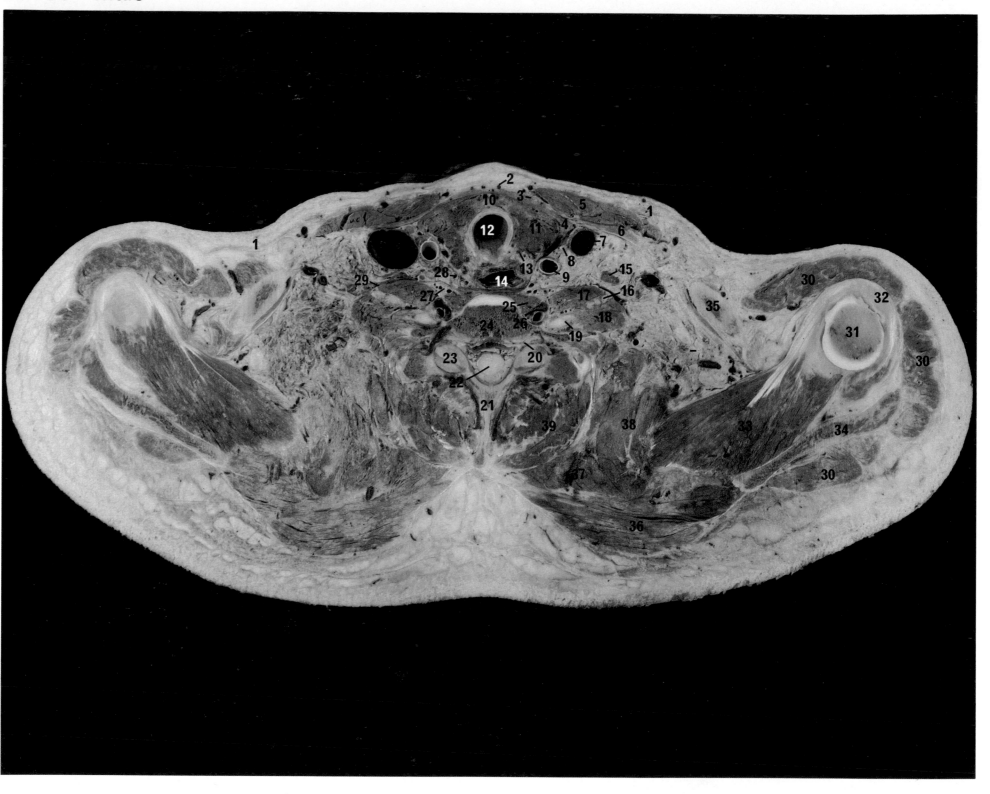

1 Platysma
2 Anterior jugular vein
3 Sternohyoid
4 Sternothyroid
5 Sternocleidomastoid
6 Omohyoid
7 Internal jugular vein
8 Vagus nerve (X)
9 Common carotid artery
10 Isthmus of thyroid gland
11 Lateral lobe of thyroid gland
12 Trachea
13 Recurrent laryngeal nerve
14 Oesophagus
15 Lymph node
16 Ventral ramus of sixth cervical nerve
17 Scalenus anterior
18 Scalenus medius
19 Ventral ramus of seventh cervical nerve
20 Dorsal root ganglion of eighth cervical nerve
21 Spine of seventh cervical vertebra – vertebra prominens
22 Spinal cord within dural sheath
23 Inferior articular facet of seventh cervical vertebra
24 Body of seventh cervical vertebra
25 Longus colli
26 Vertebral artery and vein
27 Ascending cervical artery and vein
28 Inferior thyroid artery
29 Phrenic nerve
30 Deltoid
31 Head of humerus
32 Capsule of shoulder joint
33 Supraspinatus
34 Spine of scapula
35 Coracoid process of scapula
36 Trapezius
37 Rhomboideus minor
38 Levator scapulae
39 Erector spinae

40 External jugular vein

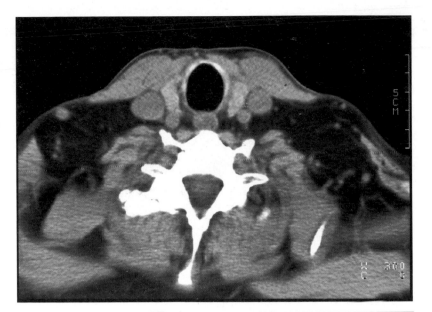

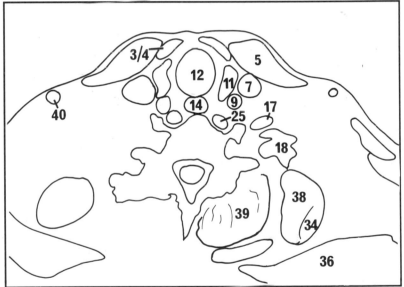

NOTES

This section traverses the body of the seventh cervical vertebra which bears the longest spine of the cervical series, the vertebra prominens (21). However, this is shorter than the spine of T1 as can easily be ascertained by feeling the back of your own neck.

Two important relationships are well demonstrated. The recurrent laryngeal nerve (13) lies in the groove between the trachea (12) and the oesophagus (14). The phrenic nerve (29) hugs the anterior aspect of the scalenus anterior (17) beneath the prevertebral fascia.

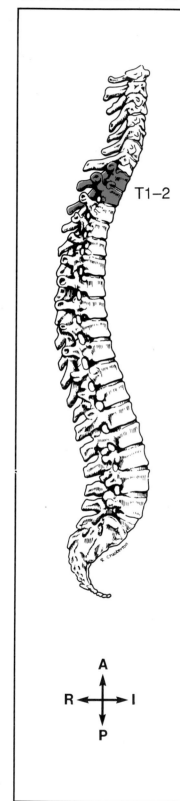

T1–2

A
R ←→ I
P

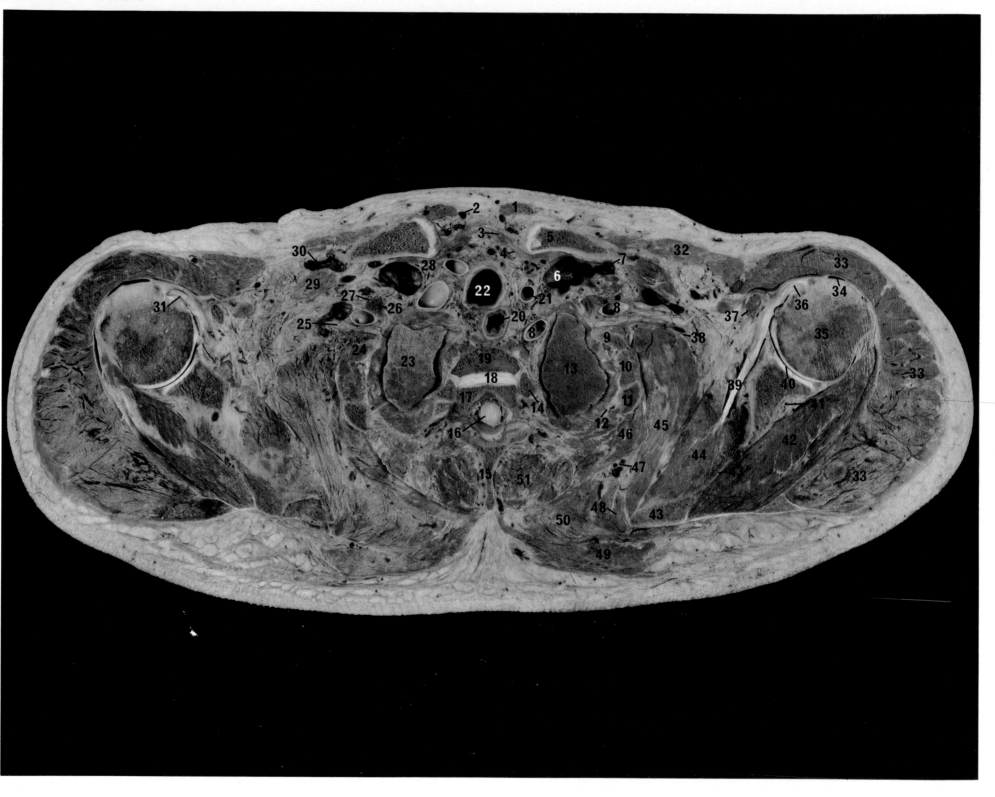

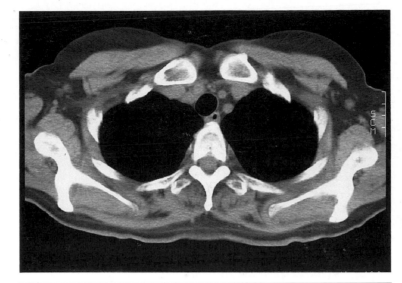

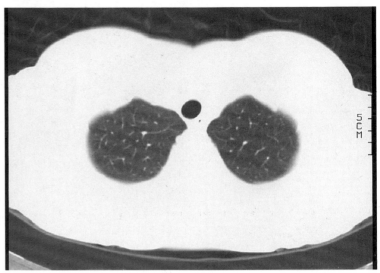

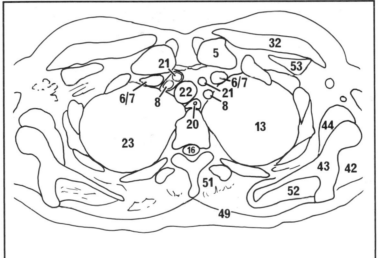

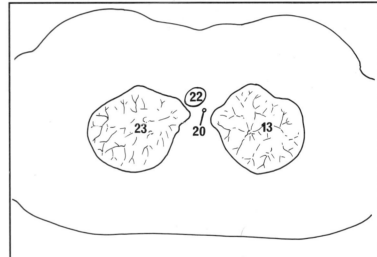

1 Sternocleidomastoid, sternal head
2 Anterior jugular vein
3 Sternohyoid
4 Sternothyroid
5 Clavicle
6 Internal jugular vein – junction with left subclavian vein
7 Left subclavian vein
8 Subclavian artery
9 First rib
10 Intercostal muscles
11 Second rib
12 Intercostal neurovascular bundle
13 Apex of left lung
14 Head of second rib
15 Spine of first thoracic vertebra
16 Spinal cord within dural sheath
17 Part of body of second thoracic vertebra
18 Part of intervertebral disc between first and second thoracic vertebrae
19 Part of body of first thoracic vertebra
20 Oesophagus
21 Common carotid artery
22 Trachea
23 Right lung apex
24 Scalenus medius
25 Root of first thoracic nerve

26 Scalenus anterior
27 Phrenic nerve
28 Vagus nerve (X)
29 Subclavius
30 Right subclavian vein
31 Tendon of right biceps long head
32 Pectoralis major
33 Deltoid
34 Subdeltoid bursa
35 Head of humerus
36 Tendon of left biceps long head
37 Coracoid process of scapula
38 Nerve to serratus anterior
39 Tendon of subscapularis
40 Glenoid fossa of scapula
41 Suprascapular artery and vein
42 Infraspinatus
43 Scapula
44 Subscapularis
45 Serratus anterior
46 Serratus posterior superior
47 Superficial (transverse) cervical artery and vein
48 Rhomboideus minor
49 Trapezius
50 Rhomboideus major
51 Erector spinae

52 Supraspinatus
53 Pectoralis minor

NOTES

This section, through the intervertebral disc between the first and second thoracic vertebrae (18), enters the apex of the thorax and traverses the apices of the upper lobes of the lungs (13, 23). There are considerable differences between the section and CT images at this level because CT is performed with the arms elevated alongside the head in order to reduce artefacts from the humeri.

Here, posterior to the medial end of the clavicle (5), the internal jugular vein (6) joins with the subclavian vein (7) to form the brachiocephalic vein (see section 32).

The intercostal neurovascular bundle (12) is well seen. Note that it comprises the intercostal vein, artery and nerve from above downwards; the nerve corresponds to the number of its overlying rib and lies protected within the subcostal groove.

Only in transverse section is the extreme thinness of the blade of the scapula (43) fully appreciated.

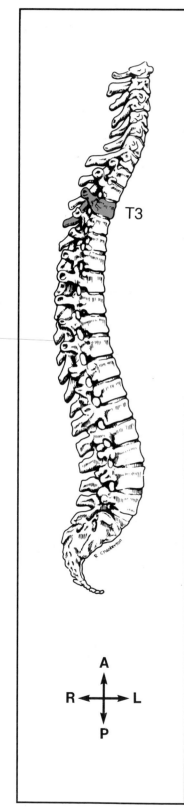

T3

A
R ← → L
P

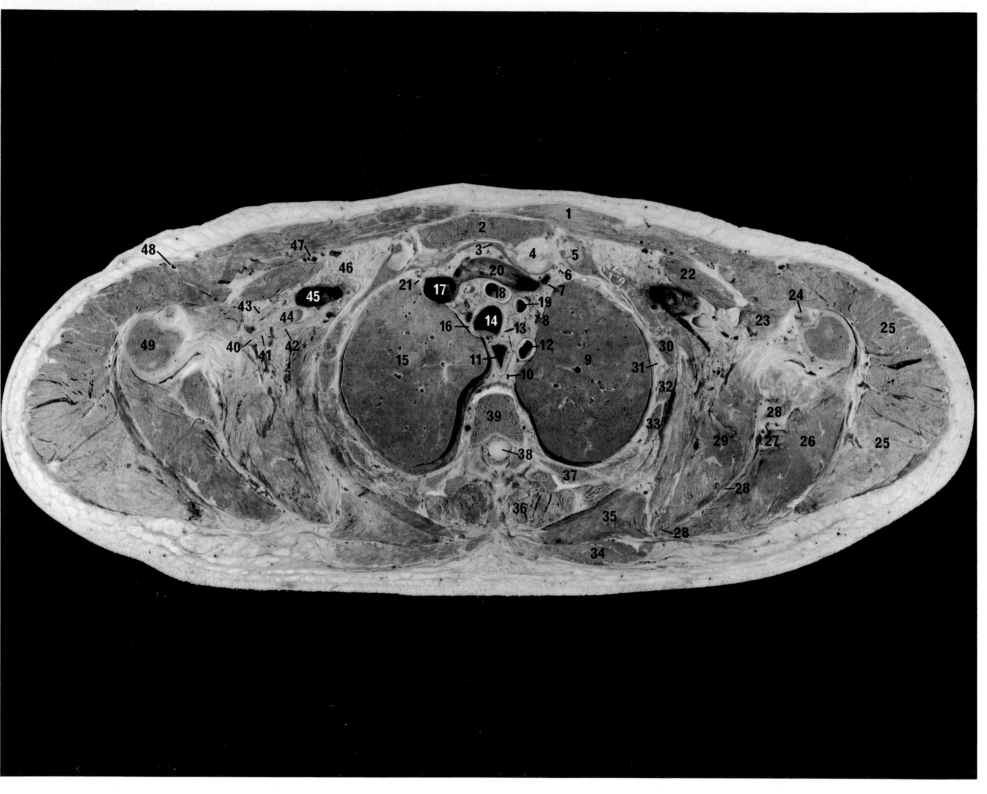

1 Pectoralis major
2 Manubrium of sternum
3 Sternothyroid
4 Sternoclavicular joint
5 First rib
6 Internal thoracic artery
7 Left phrenic nerve
8 Left vagus nerve (X)
9 Upper lobe of left lung
10 Thoracic duct
11 Oesophagus
12 Left subclavian artery
13 Left recurrent laryngeal nerve
14 Trachea
15 Upper lobe of right lung
16 Right vagus nerve (X)
17 Right brachiocephalic vein
18 Brachiocephalic artery
19 Left common carotid artery
20 Left brachiocephalic vein
21 Right phrenic nerve
22 Pectoralis minor
23 Coracobrachialis and biceps (short head)
24 Long head of biceps tendon
25 Deltoid
26 Infraspinatus
27 Suprascapular artery and vein

28 Scapula
29 Subscapularis
30 Second rib
31 Intercostal artery and vein and nerve
32 External and internal intercostal muscles
33 Third rib
34 Trapezius
35 Rhomboideus major
36 Erector spinae
37 Fourth rib with articulation of its head with body of third thoracic vertebra transverse process
38 Spinal cord within dural sheath
39 Body of third thoracic vertebra
40 Axillary nerve
41 Radial nerve
42 Ulnar nerve
43 Median nerve
44 Right axillary artery
45 Right axillary vein
46 Axillary fat
47 Pectoral branch of the acromiothoracic artery and vein
48 Cephalic vein
49 Shaft of humerus

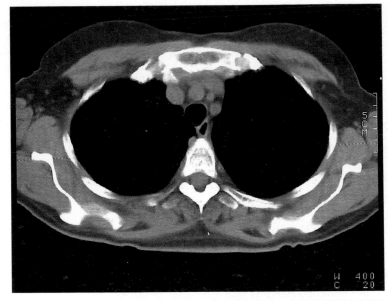

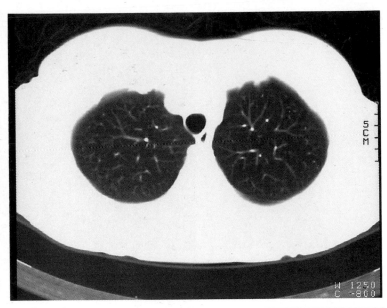

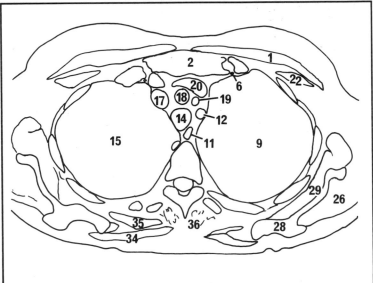

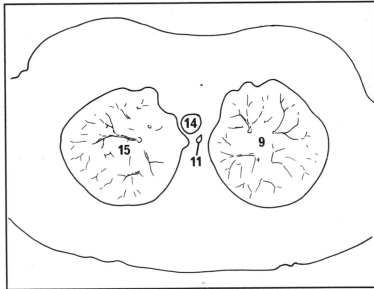

NOTES

The contents of the upper mediastinum – including oesophagus, trachea and great vessels – are demonstrated in this section, which traverses the manubrium and the third thoracic vertebra; these are also shown in section 33. This section also shows the walls and contents of the axilla.

Note that the cephalic vein (48) runs in the deltopectoral groove between the medial edge of the deltoid and the lateral edge of the pectoralis major.

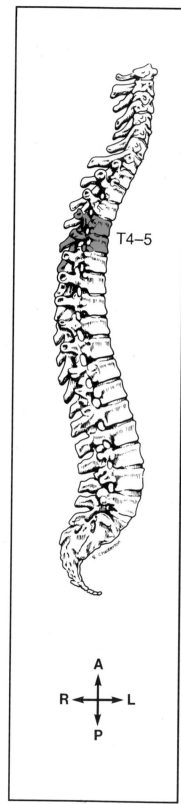

T4–5

A
R ← → L
P

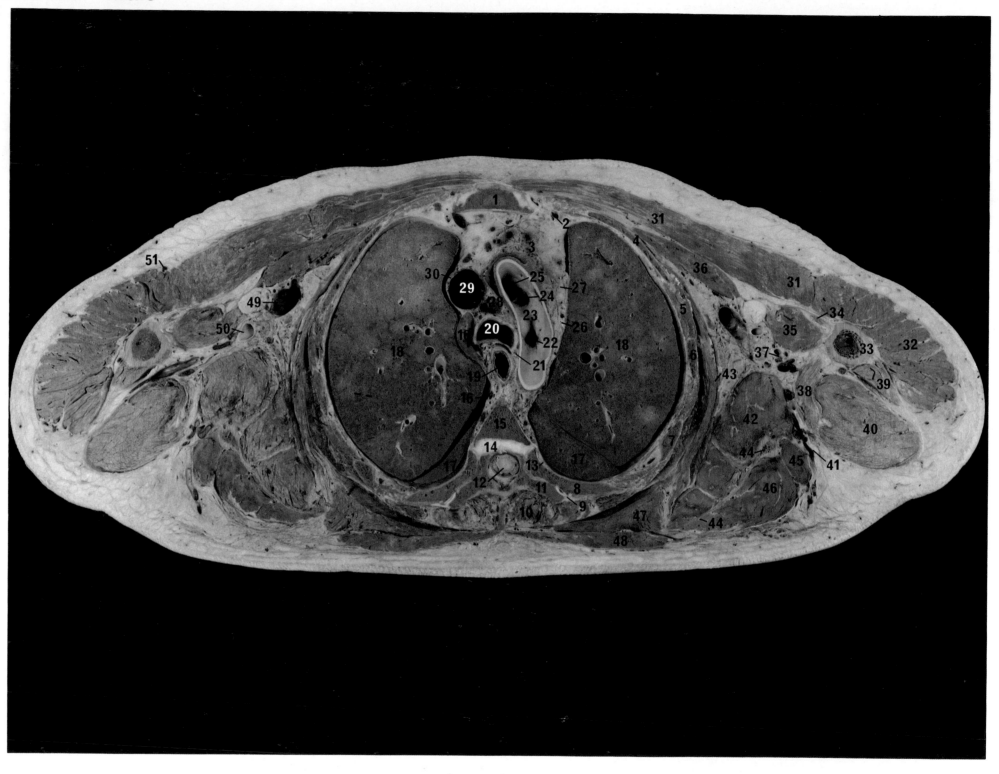

1 Manubriosternal joint (angle of Louis)
2 Internal thoracic artery and vein
3 Thymic residue within anterior mediastinal fat
4 Second rib
5 Intercostal muscles
6 Third rib
7 Fourth rib
8 Fifth rib
9 Fifth costotransverse joint
10 Erector spinae
11 Transverse process of fifth thoracic vertebra
12 Spinal cord within dural sheath
13 Sympathetic chain
14 Part of intervertebral disc between fourth and fifth thoracic vertebrae
15 Part of body of fourth thoracic vertebra
16 Azygos vein
17 Apical segment of lower lobe of lung separated by oblique fissure from (18)
18 Upper lobe of lung
19 Oesophagus
20 Trachea at bifurcation
21 Recurrent laryngeal nerve
22 Left subclavian artery orifice
23 Aortic arch
24 Left common carotid artery orifice

25 Brachiocephalic artery orifice
26 Left vagus nerve (X)
27 Left phrenic nerve
28 Pretracheal lymph node
29 Superior vena cava
30 Right phrenic nerve
31 Pectoralis major
32 Deltoid
33 Shaft of humerus
34 Biceps – long head
35 Biceps – short head and coracobrachialis
36 Pectoralis minor
37 Subscapular artery, vein and nerve
38 Latissimus dorsi
39 Triceps – lateral head
40 Triceps – long head
41 Circumflex scapular artery and vein
42 Subscapularis
43 Serratus anterior
44 Body of scapula
45 Teres minor
46 Infraspinatus
47 Rhomboideus
48 Trapezius
49 Axillary vein
50 Axillary artery
51 Cephalic vein

52 Oblique fissure

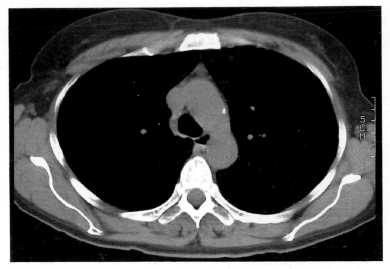
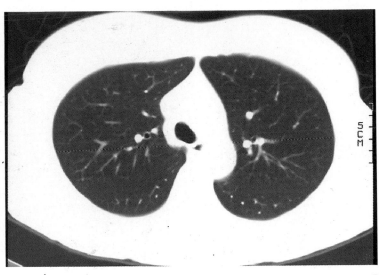
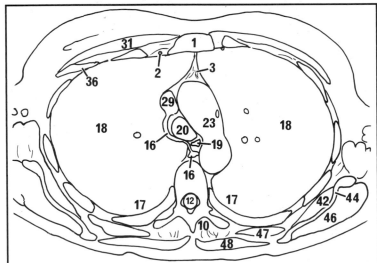
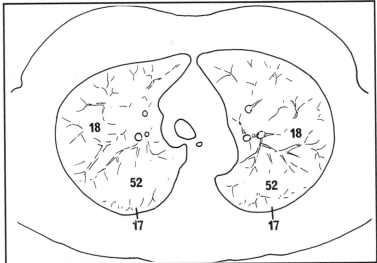

NOTES

This section passes through the important anatomical level of the manubriosternal joint, the angle of Louis (1). At this joint articulate the second costal cartilage and rib (4) and it is from here that the ribs can be conveniently counted in clinical practice. Posteriorly this plane passes through the T4/5 intervertebral disc (14).

This plane demarcates the junction between the superior mediastinum and the lower, which is subdivided into the anterior mediastinum, in front of the pericardium, the middle mediastinum, occupied by the pericardium and its contents, and the posterior mediastinum, behind the pericardium.

The trachea bifurcates at this level (20). However, in the living upright subject, the bifurcation may be as low as the level of T6, particularly in deep inspiration.

The cranial portions of the oblique fissures of the lungs (17, 52) are traversed on this section. The normal oblique fissures are often not seen on conventional CT images of the lung parenchyma. However, the position can be inferred (see CT image 33b) by the paucity of blood vessels; only small terminal vessels are present in the lung parenchyma adjacent to a fissure.

Pretracheal nodes (28) may become enlarged due to a wide variety of disease processes. They are accessible for biopsy via mediastinoscopy.

Subscapularis (42) arises not only from the periosteum of the medial two-thirds of the subscapular fossa of the scapula, but also from tendinous laminae in the muscle itself which are attached to prominent transverse ridges on the subscapular fossa. This is clearly shown in this section.

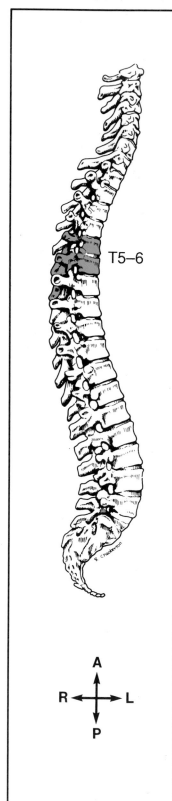

T5–6

A
R ← → L
P

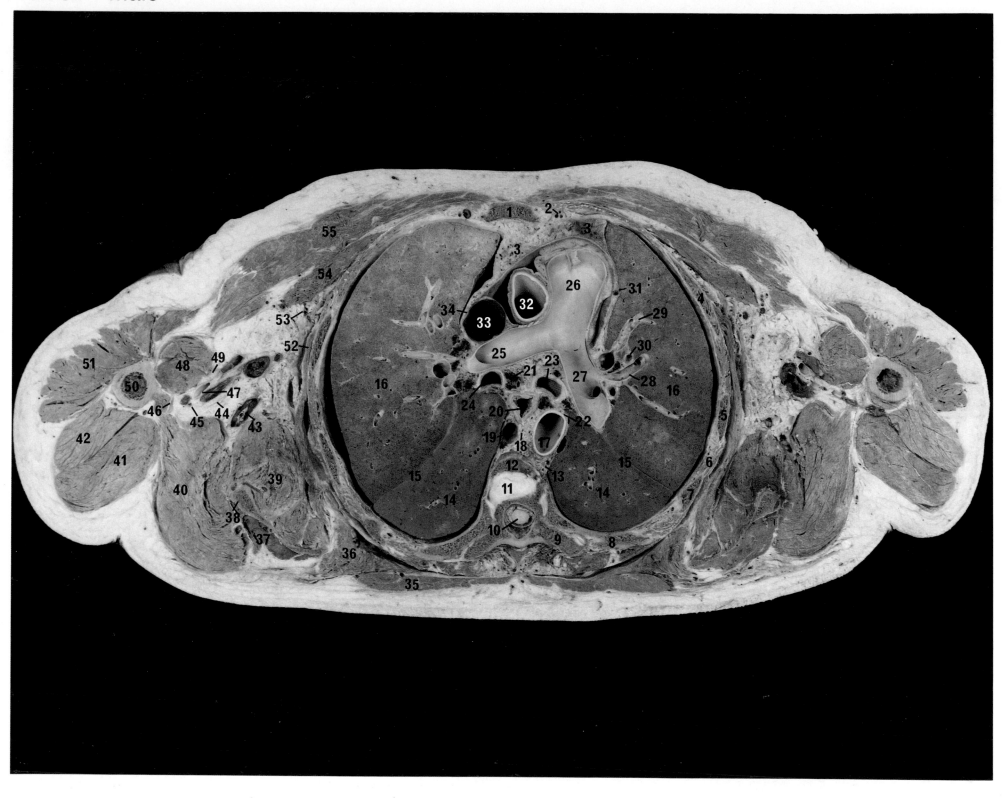

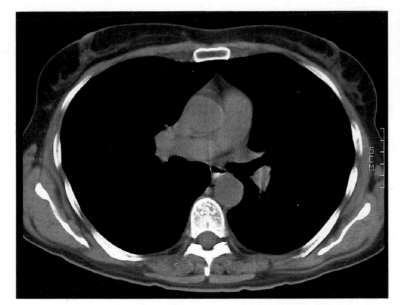

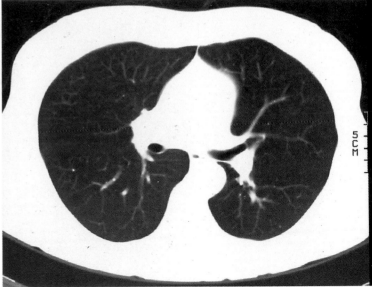

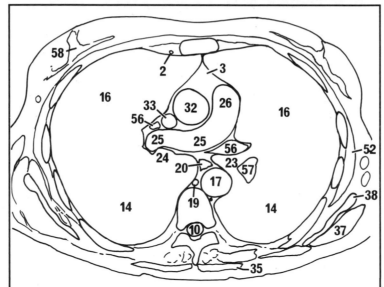

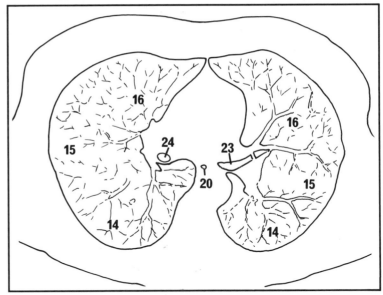

NOTES

This section, traversing the upper body of the sternum (1) and the lower part of the body of the fifth thoracic vertebra (12), passes through the great arterial trunks as these emerge from the heart, the pulmonary trunk (26) and the ascending aorta (32).

On the CT image the left main bronchus gives off its common upper lobe/lingular branch at this level. On the right, the upper lobe bronchus has already originated more cranially (on both CT images and section). Hence the term 'intermediate bronchus' (24) is applied to that portion of the right bronchus between its upper lobe and middle lobe branches.

At the left hilum the superior pulmonary vein (56) lies anterior to the bronchus (23) which lies, in turn, anterior to the left basal pulmonary artery (57). On the right side, the vein (56) lies anterior to the right pulmonary artery which lies anterior to the right intermediate bronchus (24).

In this subject, the right and left pulmonary arteries (25, 27) lie in the same axial plane. In most subjects the left pulmonary artery is at a more cranial level than the right, hence the discrepancy between the section and CT image appearances. The branches of the pulmonary artery (28) which accompany the segmental and subsegmental bronchi (30) usually lie dorsolaterally to these structures; each pulmonary segment receives an independent arterial supply. The bronchi usually separate the dorsolateral pulmonary artery branch from the ventromedially situated pulmonary vein tributary (29). Peripherally, many pulmonary venous tributaries run between, and drain adjacent, pulmonary segments. Thus an individual bronchopulmonary segment will have its own bronchus and artery but not an individual pulmonary venous drainage.

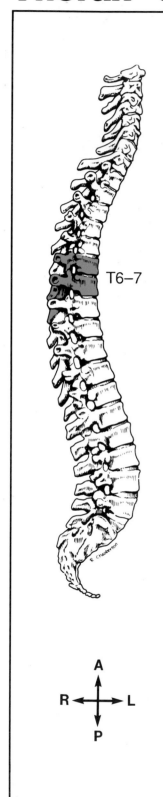

T6–7

A
R ← → L
P

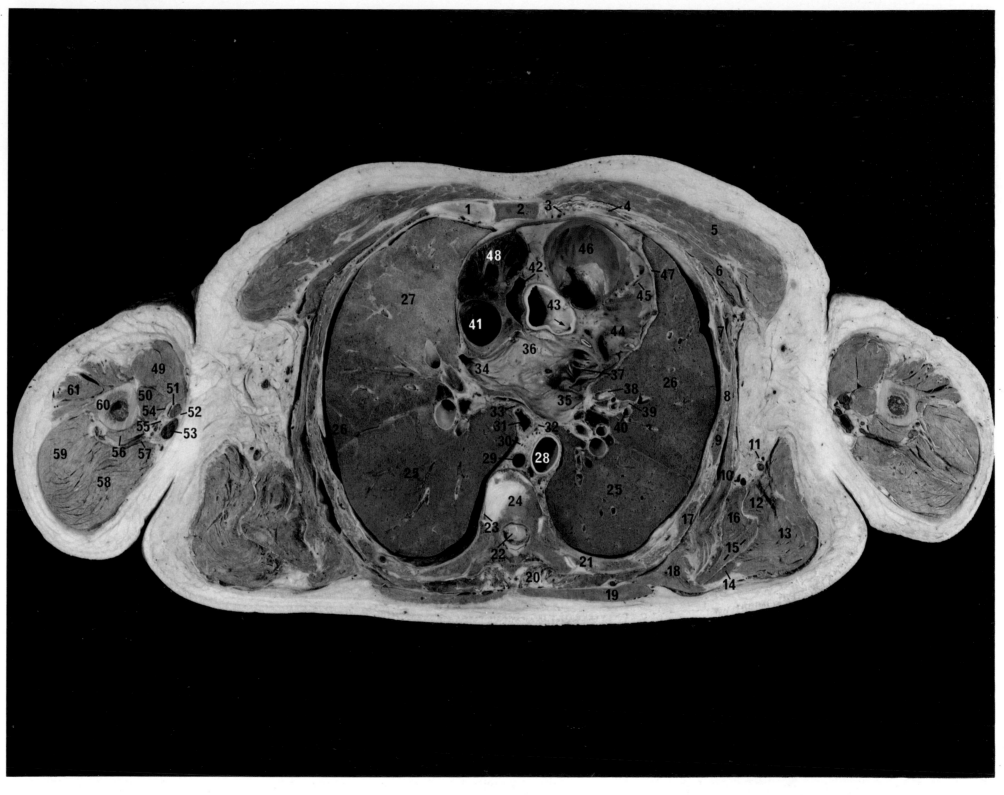

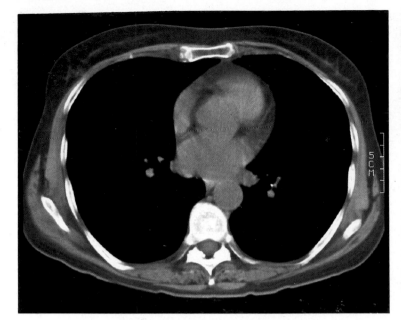

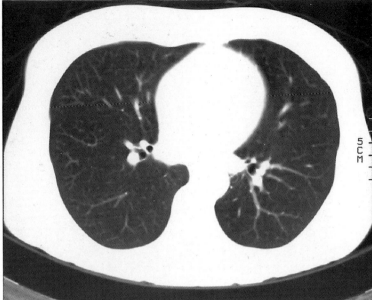

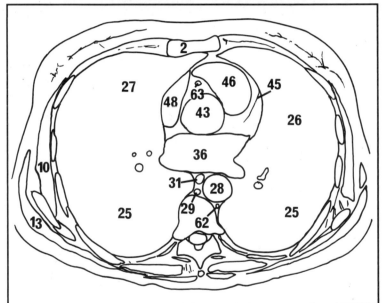

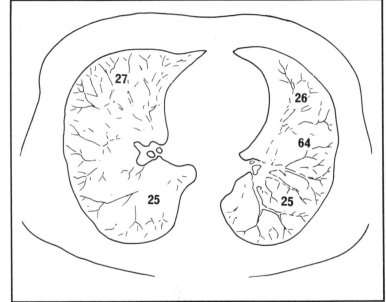

NOTES

The plane of this section traverses the lower part of the body of the sixth thoracic vertebra (24). Anteriorly it passes through the body of the sternum (2) at the level of the third costal cartilage.

The presence of a pericardial effusion in this subject has produced an artefactual gap in the superior reflection of the pericardial space (42). The aorta at its origin (43) shows the orifice of the left coronary artery. The descending aorta (28) is normally more circular in outline than in this specimen. Note that this section passes through the infundibulum of the right ventricle and demonstrates the pulmonary valves (46).

On the CT image, both the ascending aorta (43) and the region of the pulmonary valves (46) have indistinct outlines due to pulsation (compliance) of their walls during the one-second data acquisition time. (See also the ascending aorta on left-hand image, section 34.)

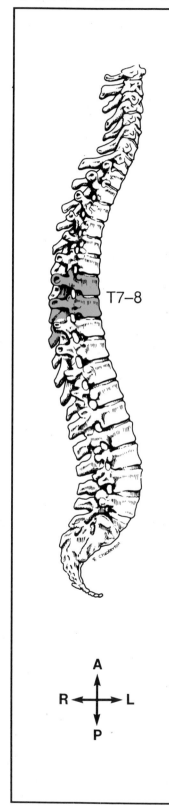

T7–8

A
R ← → L
P

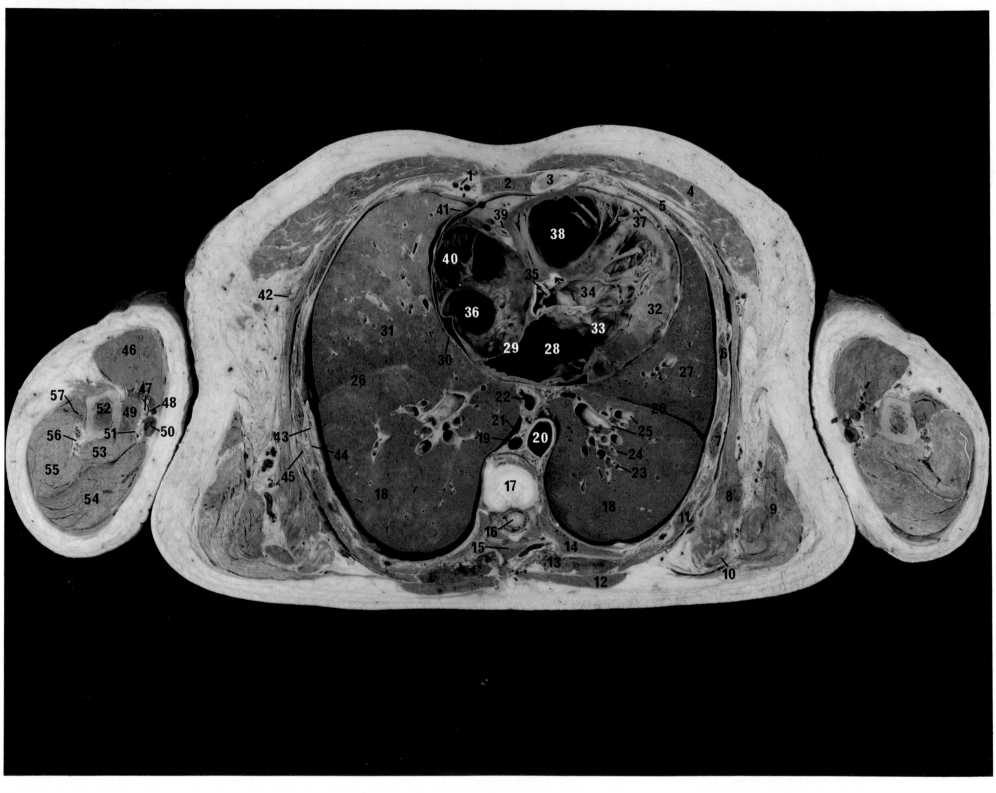

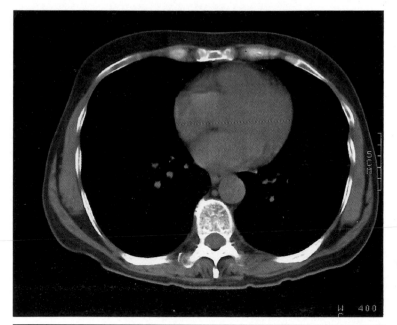

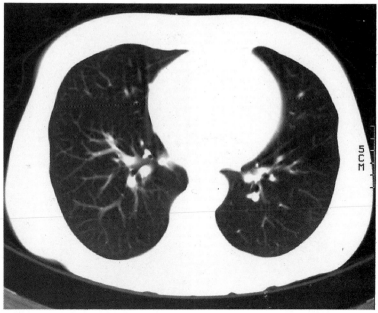

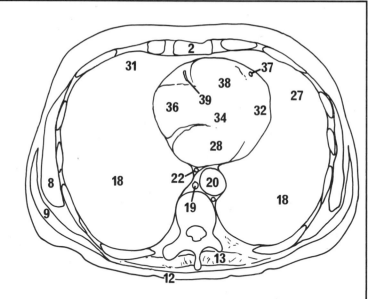

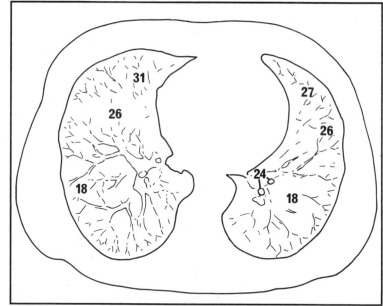

NOTES

This section lies at the level of the intervertebral disc between the seventh and eighth thoracic vertebrae (17) and passes through the body of the sternum (2) at the level of the fourth costal cartilage (3). All four cardiac chambers can be seen, and their relationships to each other appreciated. Note that the right atrium (36) forms the right border of the heart. The left atrium (28) is the major contribution to the base of the heart and lies immediately anterior to the oesophagus (22), separated by the pericardium. The left ventricle (32) forms the bulk of the left border of the heart and the right ventricle (38) constitutes the major component of the anterior cardiac surface.

In this subject, the left ventricular wall (32) becomes thinner in the region of the apex of the left ventricle due to a previous myocardial infarction.

The interatrial septum (29) has a rather curious convexity. This has been caused by extensive post-mortem thrombus in the right atrium (36). The septum is normally straighter.

The lower four or five digitations of serratus anterior (8) converge to insert on the costal aspect of the inferior angle of the scapula. This component of the muscle, together with the trapezius, powerfully pulls the inferior angle of the scapula forwards and upwards in raising the arm above the head.

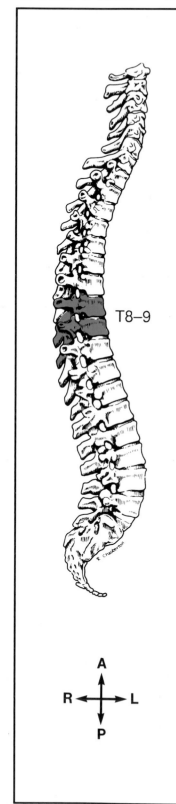

T8–9

A
R ← → L
P

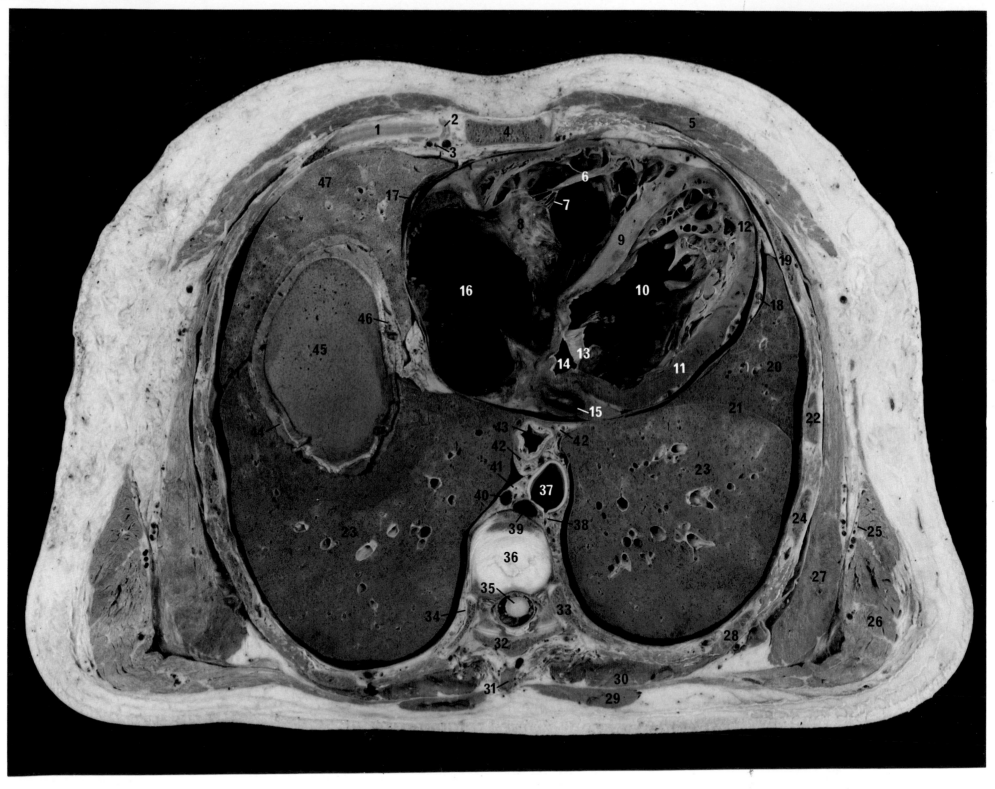

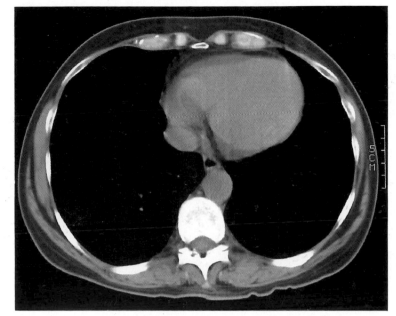
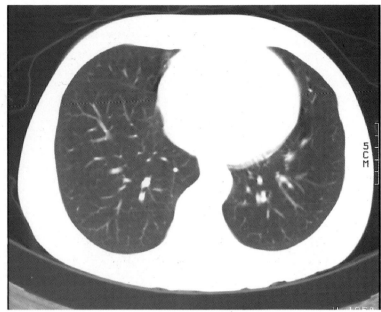
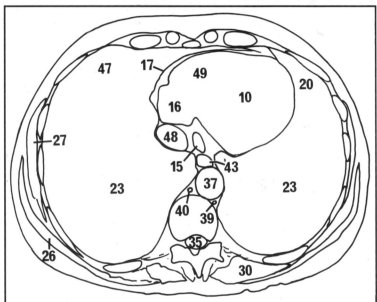
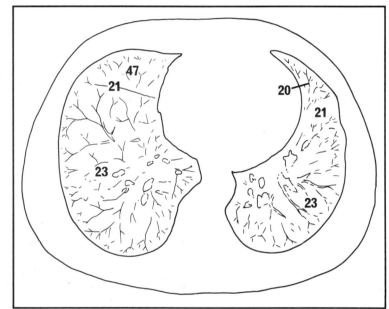

NOTES

This section traverses the intervertebral disc between the eighth and ninth thoracic vertebrae (36) and slices through the dome of the right hemidiaphragm (44) and a sliver of the underlying right lobe of the liver (45).

In this section there is considerable thinning and discoloration of the left ventricular wall at the apex (12), consistent with infarction associated with left anterior descending (interventricular) coronary arterial disease.

Note how only a tiny portion of the left atrium (14) is present on this section. This demonstrates that the left atrium is situated more cranially than the other three cardiac chambers.

The terminal fibres of the right phrenic nerve (46) usually pass through the vena caval opening in the diaphragm but may traverse the muscle itself.

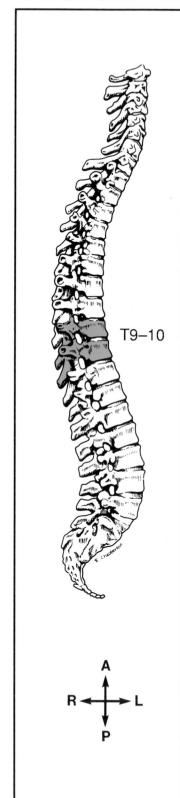

T9–10

A
R ← → L
P

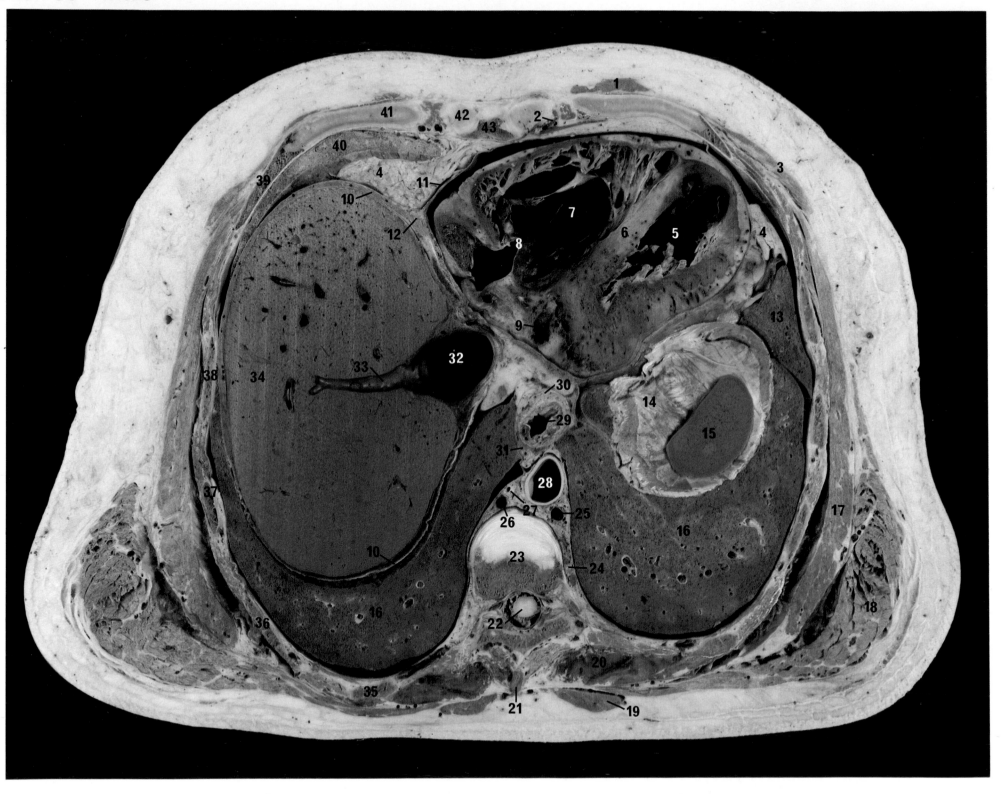

1 Pectoralis major	23 Body of ninth thoracic vertebra with part of intervertebral disc between ninth and tenth thoracic vertebrae
2 Internal thoracic artery and vein	
3 External oblique	
4 Extrapericardial pad of fat	24 Left sympathetic chain
5 Left ventricle	25 Hemiazygos vein
6 Interventricular septum	26 Azygos vein
7 Right ventricle	27 Thoracic duct
8 Tricuspid valve	28 Aorta
9 Coronary sinus	29 Oesophagus
10 Diaphragm	30 Left vagus nerve (X)
11 Fibrous pericardium	31 Right vagus nerve (X)
12 Line of fusion of diaphragm and pericardium	32 Inferior vena cava
	33 Right hepatic vein
13 Upper lobe of left lung (lingula)	34 Right lobe of liver
	35 Tenth rib
14 Left dome of diaphragm	36 Ninth rib
15 Spleen	37 Eighth rib
16 Lower lobe of lung	38 Seventh rib
17 Serratus anterior	39 Sixth rib
18 Latissimus dorsi	40 Middle lobe of right lung
19 Trapezius	41 Sixth costal cartilage
20 Erector spinae	42 Fifth costal cartilage
21 Tip of spine of eighth thoracic vertebra	43 Sternum
22 Spinal cord within dural sheath	44 Oblique fissure

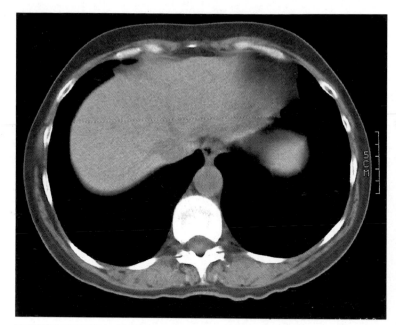
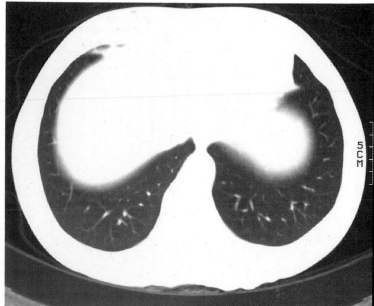

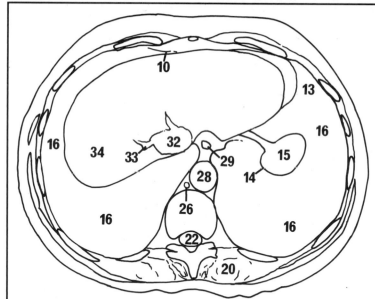
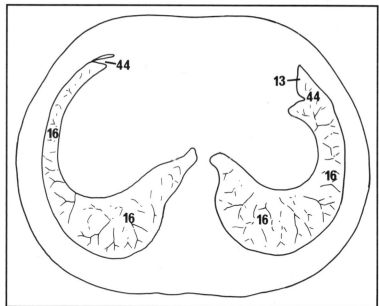

NOTES

This section is at the level of the body of the ninth thoracic vertebra (23) and traverses the left dome of the diaphragm (14). The cranial portion of the spleen (15) is therefore revealed.

The fusion of the diaphragm (10) with the base of the fibrous pericardium (11) is clearly shown at this point.

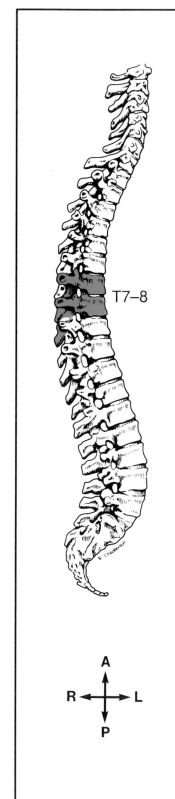

T7–8

A
R ◄─►L
P

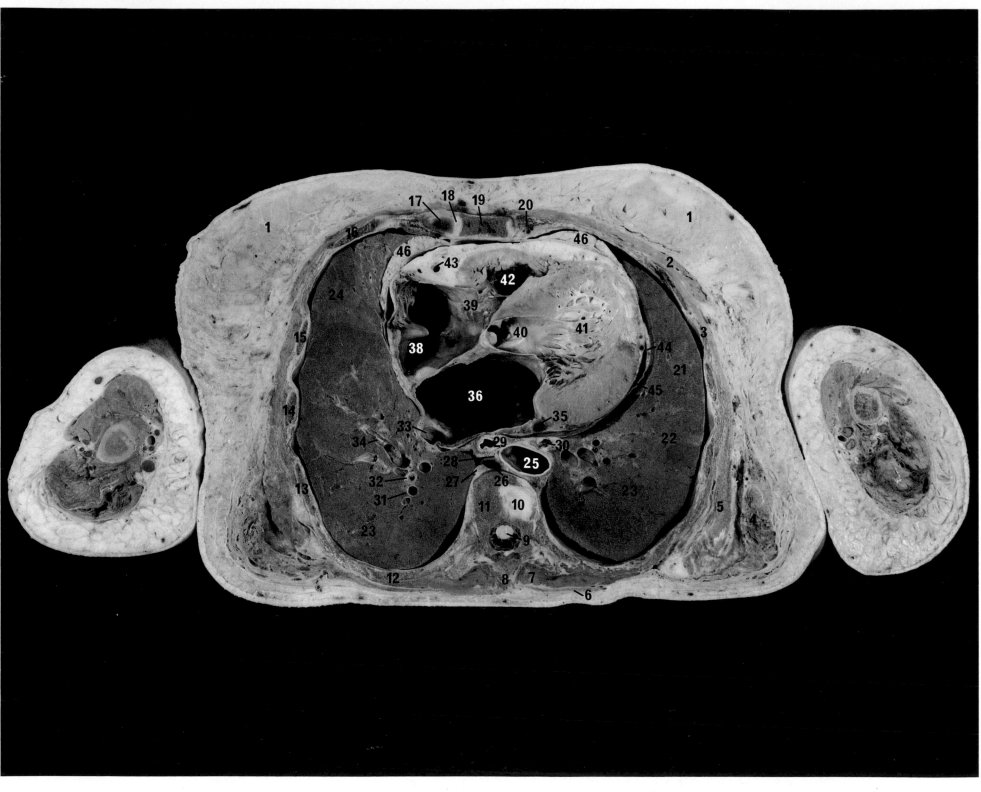

1 Breast	28 Thoracic duct
2 Pectoralis major	29 Oesophagus
3 Intercostal muscles	30 Mediastinal lymph node
4 Latissimus dorsi	31 Pulmonary arterial branch in lower lobe
5 Serratus anterior	32 Bronchus – segmental branch in lower lobe
6 Trapezius	
7 Erector spinae	
8 Spine of seventh thoracic vertebra	33 Orifice of right inferior pulmonary vein
9 Spinal cord within dural sheath	34 Right inferior pulmonary vein
10 Part of intervertebral disc between the seventh and eighth thoracic vertebrae	35 Coronary sinus
	36 Left atrium
11 Body of seventh thoracic vertebra	37 Interatrial septum
	38 Right atrium
12 Seventh rib	39 Tricuspid valve
13 Sixth rib	40 Aortic valve
14 Fifth rib	41 Left ventricle
15 Fourth rib	42 Right ventricle
16 Third rib	43 Right coronary artery
17 Third costal cartilage	44 Left phrenic nerve
18 Third sternocostal joint	45 Fibrous pericardium
19 Sternum	46 Extrapericardial fat pad
20 Internal thoracic artery and vein	47 Ascending aorta
21 Upper lobe of left lung (lingula)	48 Descending aorta
	49 Pulmonary trunk
22 Left oblique fissure	50 Right pulmonary artery
23 Lower lobe of lung	51 Superior vena cava
24 Middle lobe of right lung	52 Left basal pulmonary artery
25 Aorta	
26 Azygos vein	53 Upper lobe of right lung
27 Right sympathetic chain	54 Carcinoma right breast

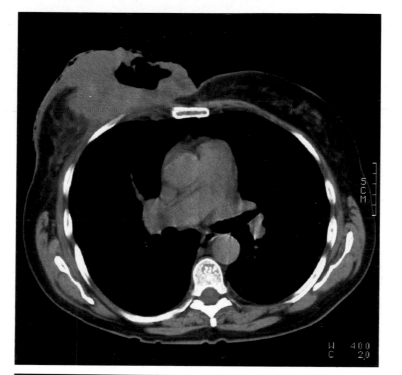

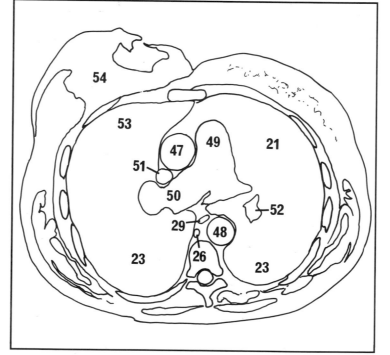

This section of a female subject passes through the body of the seventh thoracic vertebra (11) and through the third sternocostal joint (18). Note the general smaller configuration of the female thorax and the smaller, less bulky muscles.

The breast (1) contains the mammary gland. This extends vertically from the second to the sixth rib and transversely from the side of the sternum to near the mid-axillary line. The gland is situated within the superficial fascia and is separated from the fascia covering pectoralis major, serratus anterior and the external oblique muscle by loose areolar tissue. In old age, as in this specimen, the glandular tissue becomes atrophied.

This CT image shows a patient with a large carcinoma of the right breast, which has ulcerated and has extended into, and infiltrated, a wide area of adjacent skin. The anatomical level is considerably more cranial than the cadaveric section; it corresponds closely to that shown in section 34.

Note that in this section the margin of the mass of left ventricular muscle (41) has been cut across.

1　Trachea
2　Right brachiocephalic vein
3　Brachiocephalic artery
4　Left brachiocephalic vein
5　Left common carotid artery
6　Left subclavian artery
7　Manubrium of sternum
9　Internal thoracic artery and vein
10　Pectoralis major
11　Pectoralis minor
16　Oesophagus
19　Right superior intercostal vein
20　Fat in pretracheal space

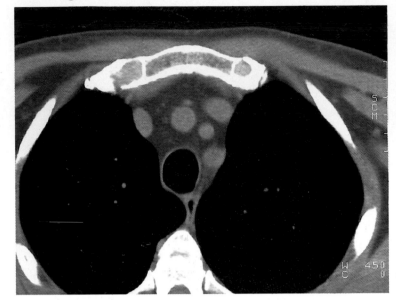
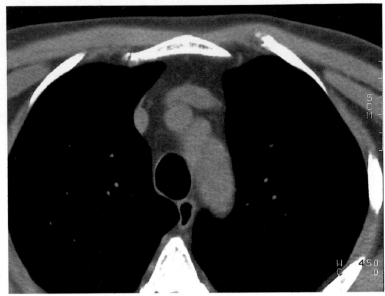
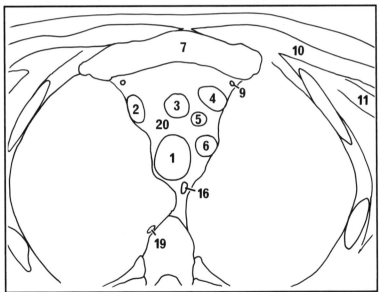
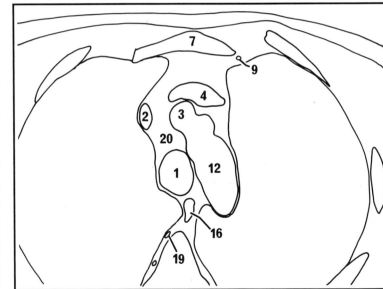

NOTES

This patient has copious mediastinal fat which makes the normal structures very conspicuous. Enlarged lymph nodes would show up well in such a patient (see section 34). If such nodes lie in the pretracheal space (20), biopsy material can be obtained via mediastinoscopy.

The trachea (1) is bifurcating on image 4; this point is known as the carina. The left pulmonary artery (15) lies at a more cranial level than the right: it is just entering part of the section shown on image

4. It appears indistinct because only part of the thickness of the slice is occupied by this structure ('partial volume' effect). The space immediately caudal to the aortic arch and cranial to the bifurcation of the pulmonary artery is known as the subaortic fossa or aortopulmonary window. The ligamentum arteriosum (the obliterated ductus arteriosus passing from the left pulmonary artery to the aorta) runs through this space. This fossa may also contain enlarged lymph nodes.

1 Trachea
2 Right brachiocephalic vein
4 Left brachiocephalic vein
7 Manubrium of sternum
8 Body of sternum
9 Internal thoracic artery and vein
10 Pectoralis major
11 Pectoralis minor
12 Aortic arch (with fleck of calcification in wall on image 3)
13 Ascending aorta
14 Descending aorta
15 Left pulmonary artery
16 Oesophagus
17 Superior vena cava
18 Azygos vein
19 Right superior intercostal vein
20 Fat in pretracheal space
21 Fat in anterior mediastinal space (with thymic remnant)
22 Azygos – oesophageal recess

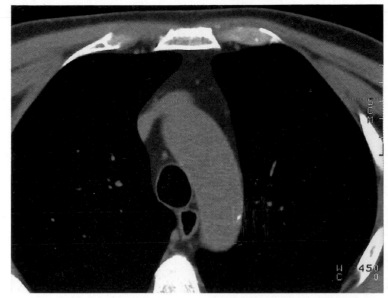
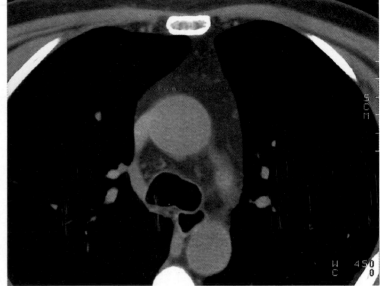

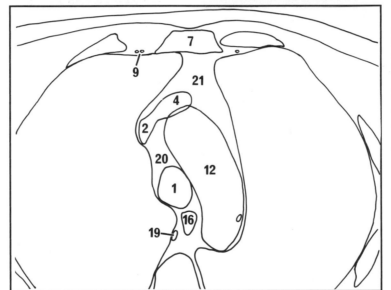
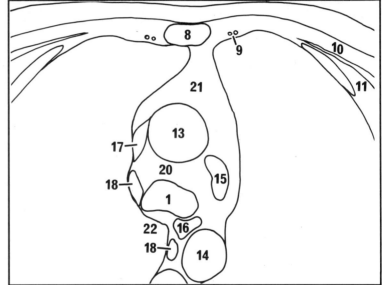

NOTES

This patient has copious mediastinal fat which makes the normal structures very conspicuous. Enlarged lymph nodes would show up well in such a patient (see section 34). If such nodes lie in the pretracheal space (20), biopsy material can be obtained via mediastinoscopy.

The trachea (1) is bifurcating on image 4; this point is known as the carina. The left pulmonary artery (15) lies at a more cranial level than the right: it is just entering part of the section shown on image

4. It appears indistinct because only part of the thickness of the slice is occupied by this structure ('partial volume' effect). The space immediately caudal to the aortic arch and cranial to the bifurcation of the pulmonary artery is known as the subaortic fossa or aortopulmonary window. The ligamentum arteriosum (the obliterated ductus arteriosus passing from the left pulmonary artery to the aorta) runs through this space. This fossa may also contain enlarged lymph nodes.

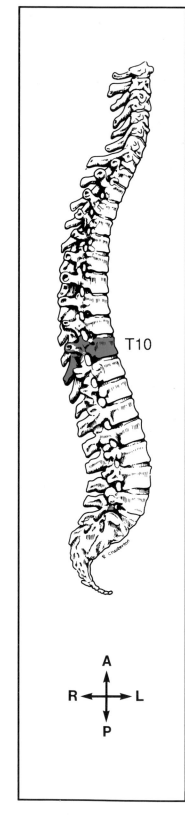

T10

A
R ← → L
P

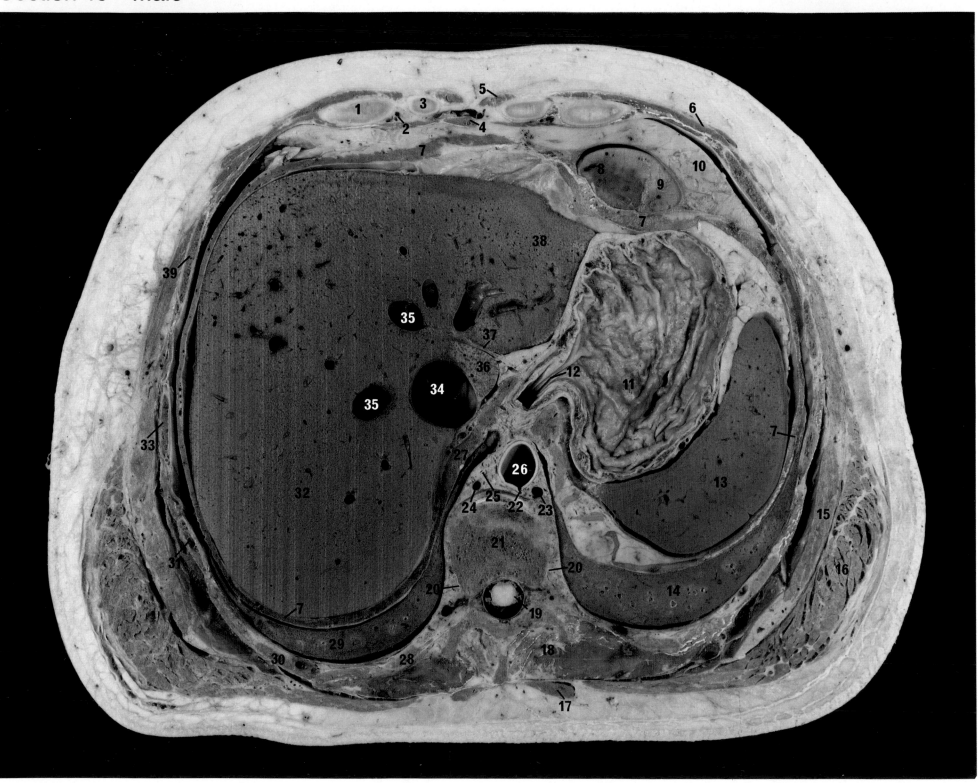

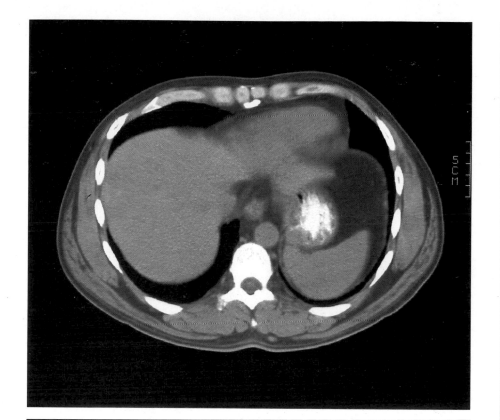

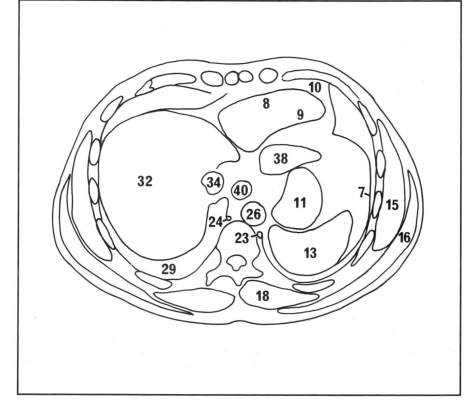

NOTES

This section passes through the body of the tenth thoracic vertebra (21) and anteriorly transects the xiphoid (4).

The oesophagogastric junction (12) is seen in longitudinal section. This acts as a physiological sphincter in the prevention of reflux. The fundus of the stomach (11) contains air in the erect position but in the supine position is normally full of fluid. It is opaque in the CT image because of the ingested radio-opaque iodinated material.

The lesser omentum is the fold of peritoneum which extends to the liver from the lesser curvature of the stomach and the commencement of the duodenum. Superiorly it attaches to the porta hepatis and to the bottom of the fissure for the ligamentum venosum (37). At the cranial margin of this fissure, the lesser omentum reaches the diaphragm, where its two layers separate to surround the lower end of the oesophagus.

The ligamentum venosum is the thrombosed cord of the ductus venosus which, in fetal life, connects the left portal vein to the anterior aspect of the inferior vena cava.

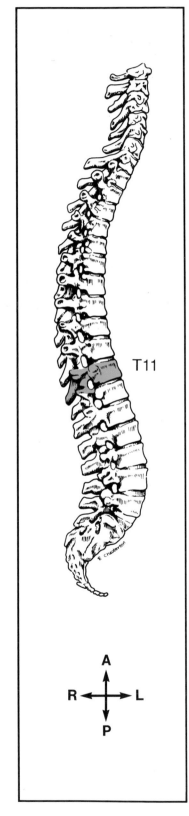

T11

A
R ← → L
P

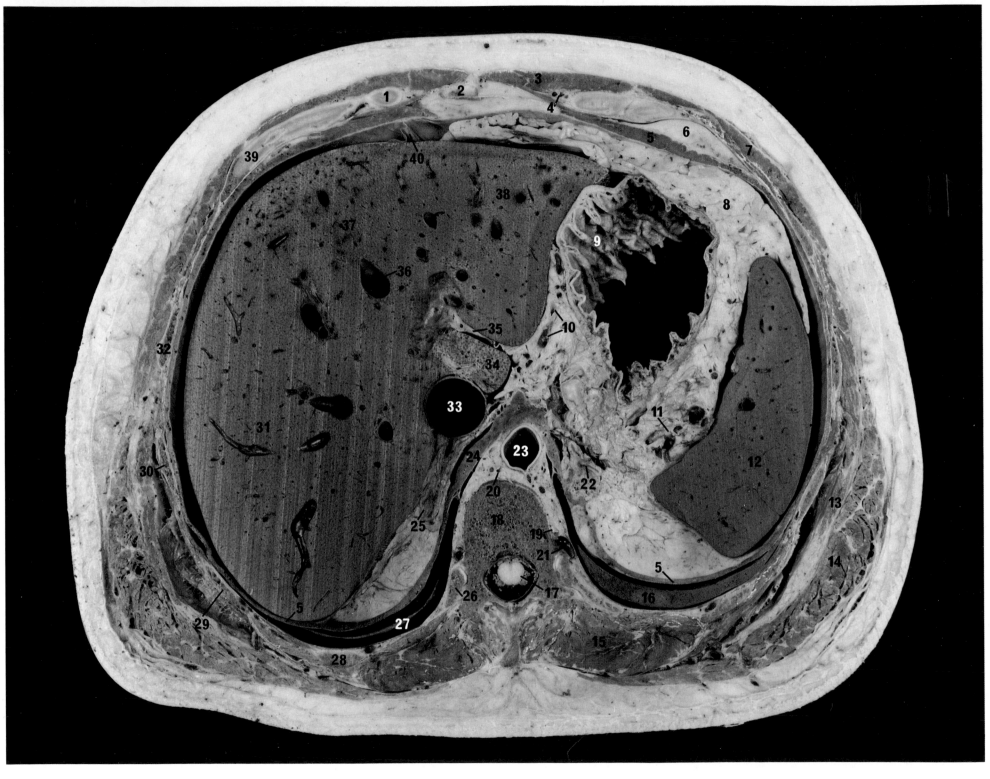

1 Seventh costal cartilage
2 Xiphoid
3 Rectus abdominis
4 Superior epigastric artery and vein
5 Diaphragm
6 Pericardial fat
7 External oblique
8 Greater omentum
9 Body of stomach
10 Left gastric artery branches
11 Splenic pedicle
12 Spleen
13 External oblique
14 Latissimus dorsi
15 Erector spinae
16 Lower lobe of left lung
17 Spinal cord within dural sheath
18 Body of eleventh thoracic vertebra
19 Intercostal artery
20 Thoracic duct
21 Intercostal vein
22 Left suprarenal gland
23 Aorta
24 Right crus of diaphragm

25 Right suprarenal gland
26 Head of eleventh rib
27 Lower lobe of right lung
28 Tenth rib
29 Ninth rib
30 Eighth rib
31 Right lobe of liver
32 Seventh rib
33 Inferior vena cava
34 Caudate lobe of liver
35 Lesser omentum in fissure for ligamentum venosum
36 Hepatic vein
37 Left lobe of liver medial segment
38 Left lobe of liver lateral segment
39 Sixth costal cartilage and rib
40 Falciform ligament

41 Portal vein
42 Pancreas
43 Left colic (splenic) flexure
44 Splenic vein
45 Left crus of diaphragm
46 Median arcuate ligament

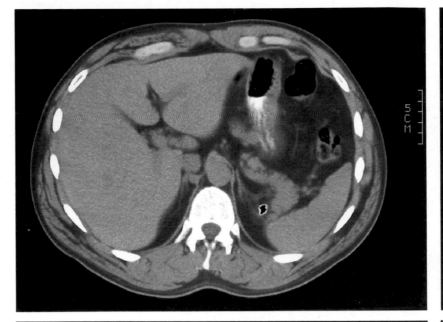

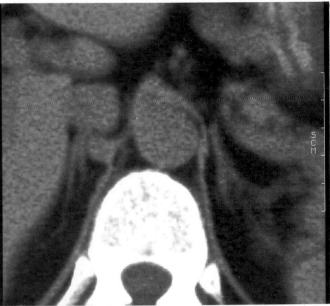

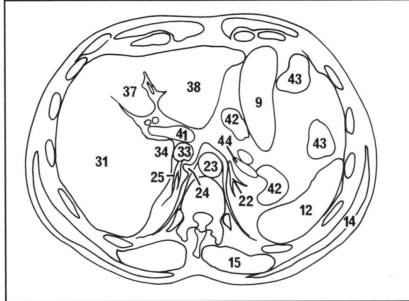

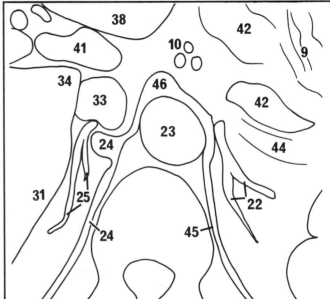

NOTES

This section passes through the body of the eleventh thoracic vertebra (18) and the xiphoid (2).

This is the most caudal section which transects intrathoracic viscera – note the pericardial fat anteriorly (6) and lower lobe of the left lung (16).

The suprarenal glands (22, 25) have a constant relationship to the diaphragmatic crura (24, 45). Note on the CT images that the separate limbs of the suprarenal glands are demarcated.

The right crus of the diaphragm (24) on the CT image is often bulky. The crura change shape during respiration; normally they are bulkier on inspiration.

On the CT image the pancreas (42) is just visible as it enters the plane of this section. It is better seen in more caudal sections. As the pancreas occupies only part of the section, its outlines are not sharply demarcated. This is another example of the 'partial volume' effect.

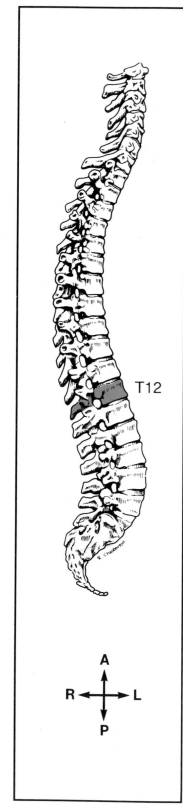

T12

A
R ← → L
P

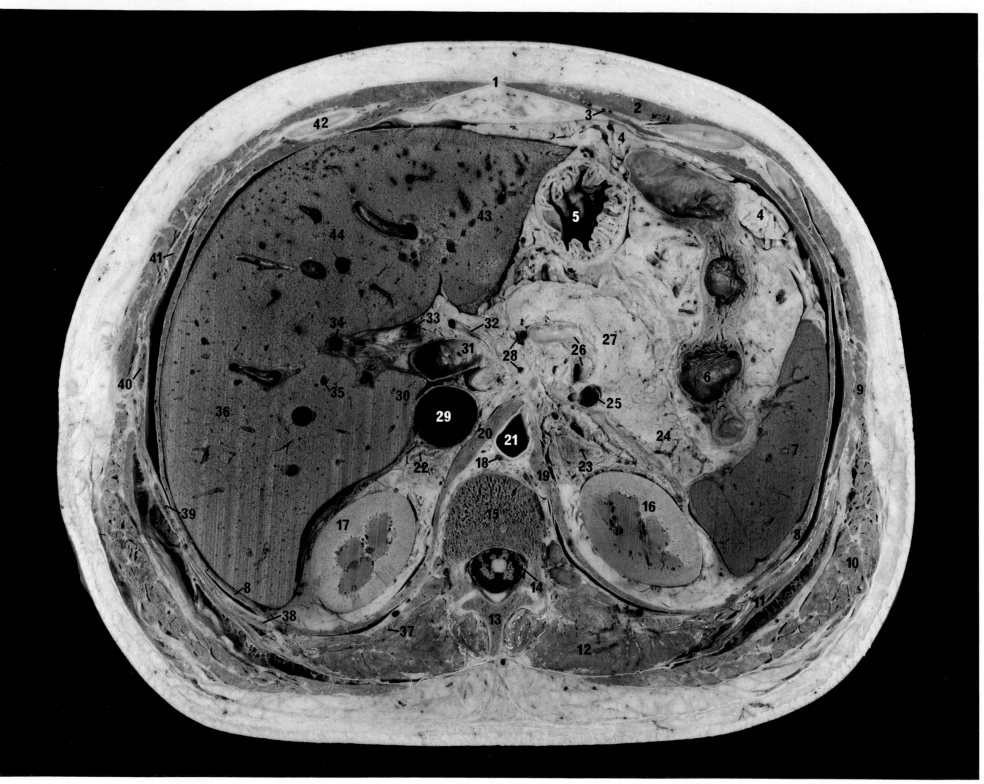

1 Linea alba
2 Rectus abdominis
3 Superior epigastric artery and vein
4 Greater omentum
5 Body of stomach
6 Left colic (splenic) flexure
7 Spleen
8 Diaphragm
9 External oblique
10 Latissimus dorsi
11 Serratus posterior inferior
12 Erector spinae
13 Spine of eleventh thoracic vertebra
14 Conus medullaris surrounded by cauda equina within dural sheath
15 Body of twelfth thoracic vertebra
16 Left kidney
17 Right kidney
18 Thoracic duct
19 Left crus of diaphragm
20 Right crus of diaphragm
21 Aorta
22 Right suprarenal gland
23 Left suprarenal gland
24 Tail of pancreas

25 Splenic vein
26 Splenic artery
27 Body of pancreas
28 Left gastric artery and vein
29 Inferior vena cava
30 Caudate lobe of liver
31 Portal vein
32 Hepatic artery
33 Common bile duct
34 Radicle of portal vein
35 Hepatic artery branch
36 Right lobe of liver
37 Twelfth rib
38 Eleventh rib
39 Tenth rib
40 Ninth rib
41 Eighth rib
42 Seventh costal cartilage
43 Left lobe of liver (lateral segment)
44 Left lobe of liver (medial segment)

45 Gall bladder
46 Ligamentum teres
47 Jejunum

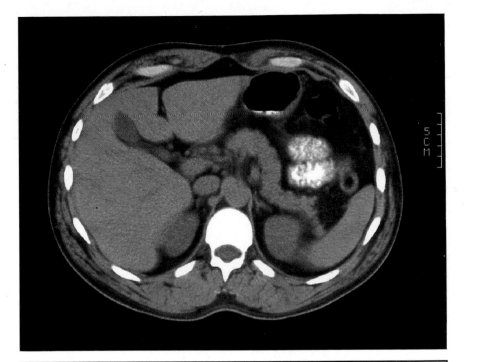

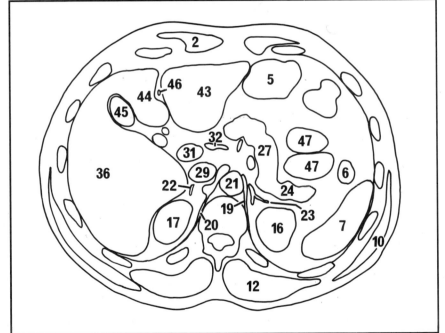

NOTES

This section passes through the body of the twelfth thoracic vertebra (15). It demonstrates well the relationships of the structures at the porta hepatis – the common bile duct (33) anterior and to the right, the hepatic artery (32) anterior and to the left and the portal vein (31) posterior to these structures. The inferior vena cava (29) lies immediately behind the portal vein: between the two is the epiploic foramen, or the aditus to the lesser sac (the foramen of Winslow). The division between the cortex (peripheral) and medulla (central) of the kidneys (16, 17) is well shown: in the plane of this division run the small arcuate vessels which can just be identified in this section. Post mortem changes account for the discrepancy in the differentiation between cortex and medulla in the left kidney.

A Note on the lobes of the liver

The gross *anatomical division* of the liver is into a right and left lobe, demarcated by the attachment of the falciform ligament on the anterior surface and by the fissures for the ligamentum teres and ligamentum venosum on the visceral surface. This is simply a gross anatomical descriptive term with no morphological significance. Two subsidiary additional lobes are marked out on the visceral aspect of the liver – the quadrate lobe anteriorly, between the gall bladder fossa and the fissure for the ligamentum teres, and the caudate lobe posteriorly between the groove for the inferior vena cava and the fissure for the ligamentum venosum. The transverse fissure for the porta hepatis separates the quadrate and caudate lobes.

The distribution of the right and left branches of the hepatic artery and of the hepatic duct show that the *morphological division* of the liver is into a right and left lobe demarcated by a plane which passes through the fossa of the gall bladder and the fossa of the inferior vena cava (the median plane of the liver). Morphologically, the quadrate lobe and left half of the caudate lobe are part of the morphological left lobe of the liver.

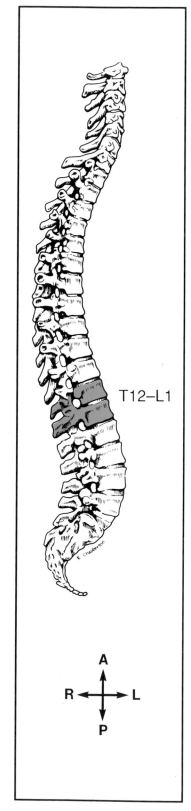

T12–L1

A
R ← → L
P

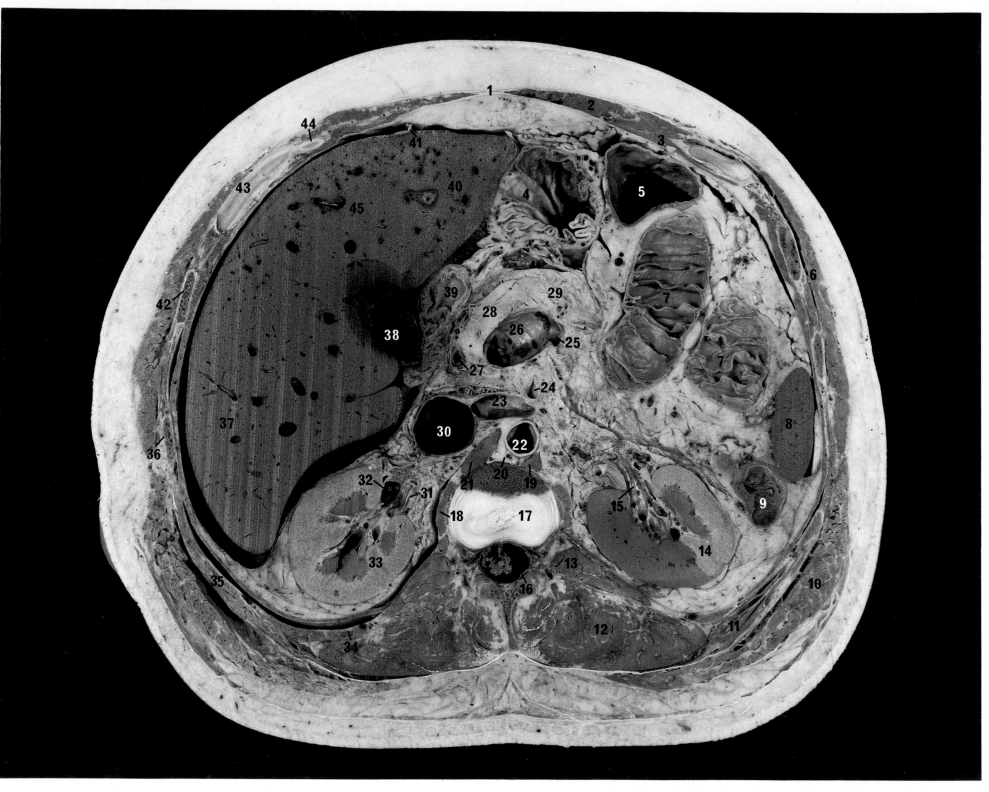

1 Linea alba
2 Rectus abdominis
3 Transversus abdominis
4 Stomach, body/antrum
5 Transverse colon
6 External oblique
7 Jejunum
8 Lower pole of spleen
9 Descending colon
10 Latissimus dorsi
11 Serratus posterior inferior
12 Erector spinae
13 Quadratus lumborum
14 Left kidney
15 Left renal vein (intrarenal portion) – see also (23)
16 Conus medullaris surrounded by cauda equina within dural sheath
17 Part of intervertebral disc between the twelfth thoracic and first lumbar vertebra with part of body of twelfth thoracic vertebra
18 Psoas major
19 Left crus of diaphragm
20 Cisterna chyli
21 Right crus of diaphragm
22 Aorta

23 Left renal vein
24 Superior mesenteric artery
25 Splenic vein
26 Portal vein (commencement)
27 Common bile duct
28 Head of pancreas
29 Neck of pancreas
30 Inferior vena cava
31 Right renal artery
32 Right renal vein
33 Right kidney
34 Twelfth rib
35 Eleventh rib
36 Tenth rib
37 Right lobe of liver
38 Gall bladder
39 First part of duodenum (cap)
40 Left lobe of liver (lateral segment)
41 Falciform ligament
42 Ninth rib
43 Eighth costal cartilage
44 Ninth costal cartilage
45 Left lobe of liver (medial segment)

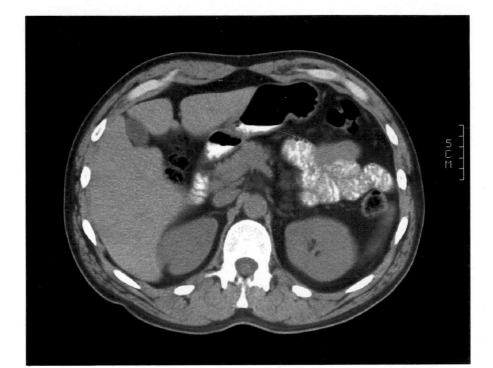

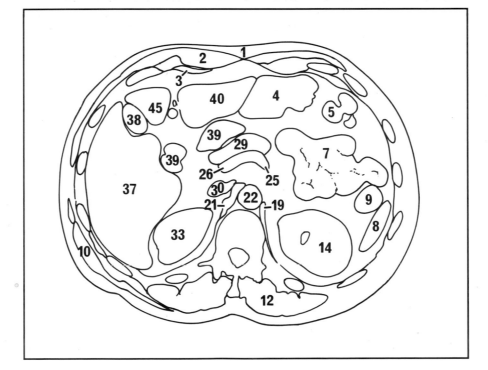

NOTES

This section transects the intervertebral disc between the twelfth thoracic and the first lumbar vertebra (17). The spinal cord tapers into the conus medullaris (16) which terminates, in this subject, at the level of the body of the first lumbar vertebra. The site of termination is variable, the range being from the disc between the twelfth thoracic and first lumbar vertebra to the lower border of the second lumbar vertebra.

The plane of this section passes through the left renal vein (23) and demonstrates well the close relationship of this vein to the superior mesenteric artery (24), which passes forward from its aortic origin (22) immediately superior to the vein. These features are well demonstrated on the CT image, section 44.

Note the circular folds of mucous membrane which project into the lumen of the small intestine transversely to its long axis (7). These are termed the *plicae circulares*. Radiologists and clinicians refer to them as *valvulae conniventes*.

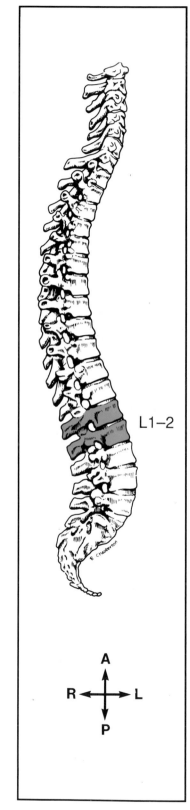

L1–2

A
R ←→ L
P

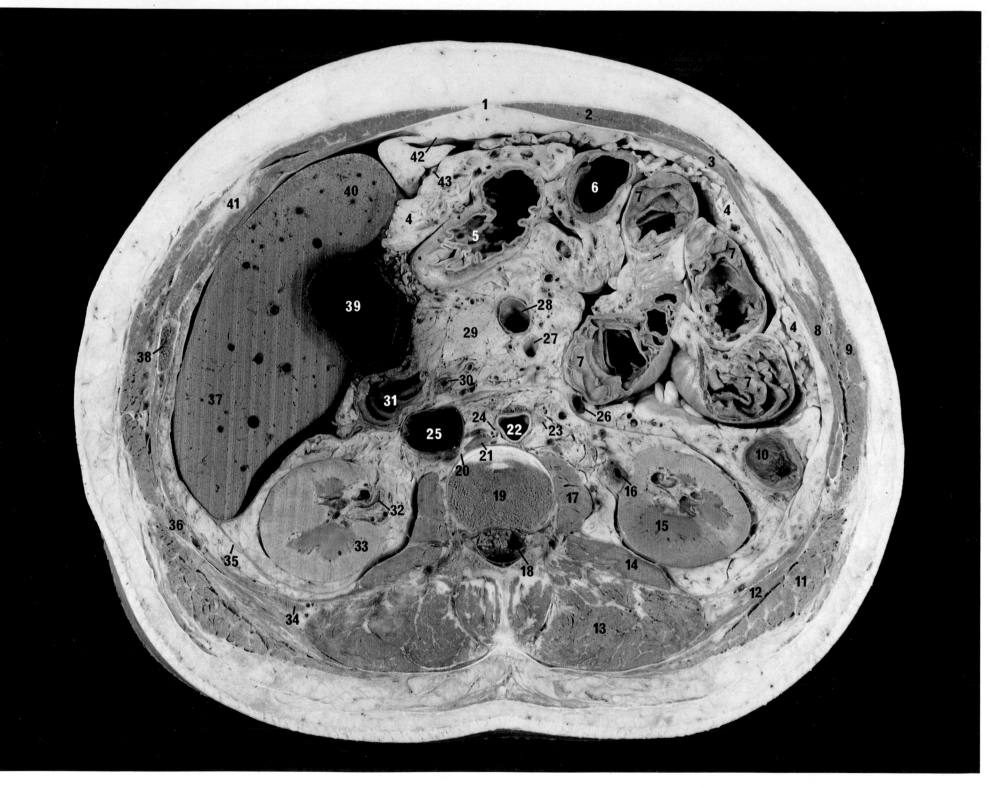

1 Linea alba	23 Para-aortic lymph node
2 Rectus abdominis	24 Cisterna chyli
3 Transversus abdominis	25 Inferior vena cava
4 Greater omentum	26 Inferior mesenteric vein
5 Antrum of stomach	27 Superior mesenteric artery
6 Transverse colon	28 Superior mesenteric vein
7 Jejunum	29 Head of pancreas
8 Internal oblique	30 Common bile duct
9 External oblique	31 Duodenum
10 Descending colon	32 Commencement of right ureter
11 Latissimus dorsi	33 Right kidney
12 Serratus posterior inferior	34 Twelfth rib
13 Erector spinae	35 Renal fascia
14 Quadratus lumborum	36 Eleventh rib
15 Left kidney	37 Right lobe of liver
16 Left ureter	38 Tenth rib
17 Psoas major	39 Gall bladder
18 Cauda equina within dural sheath	40 Left lobe of liver (medial segment)
19 Body of first lumbar vertebra with portion of intervertebral disc between the first and second lumbar vertebrae	41 Ninth costal cartilage
	42 Falciform ligament
20 Right sympathetic chain	43 Left lobe of liver (lateral segment)
21 Right crus of diaphragm	
22 Aorta	44 Left renal vein

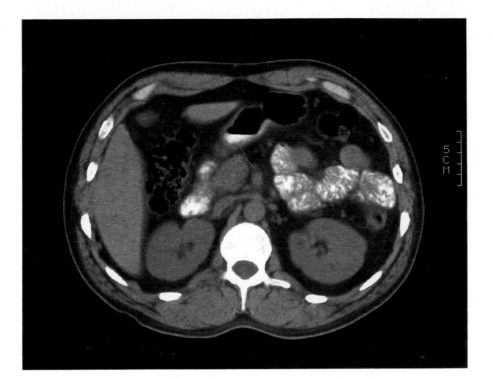

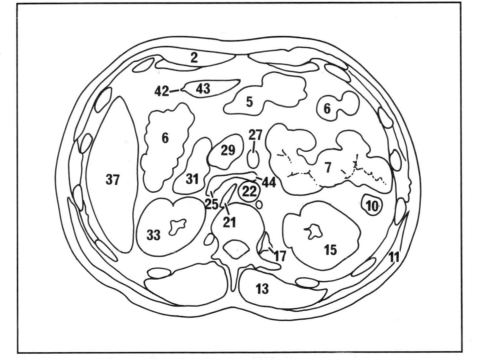

NOTES

This section passes through the body of the first lumbar vertebra (19) with a small portion of the intervertebral disc between the first and second lumbar vertebrae.

Both in this section and in the CT image the loops of jejunum (7) are fractionally wider than normal. Not all the small bowel loops in the CT image have been uniformly opacified by the ingested iodinated material.

The kidneys (15, 33) are embedded in a mass of fatty connective tissue termed the perirenal (perinephric) fat, which is thickest at their medial and lateral borders. The fibro-areolar tissue surrounding the kidney and perirenal fat condenses to form a sheath termed the renal fascia (35). At the lateral border of the kidney the two layers of the renal fascia are fused. The anterior layer is carried medially in front of the kidney and its vessels and merges with the connective tissue in front of the aorta and inferior vena cava. The posterior layer extends medially in front of the fascia covering quadratus lumborum (14) and psoas major (17) and to the vertebrae and intervertebral discs. The perirenal fat and renal fascia are surrounded by further retroperitoneal (pararenal) fatty connective tissue. The amount will vary with the relative obesity of the subject.

In this section a tiny portion of the lateral segment of the left lobe of the liver can be seen (43).

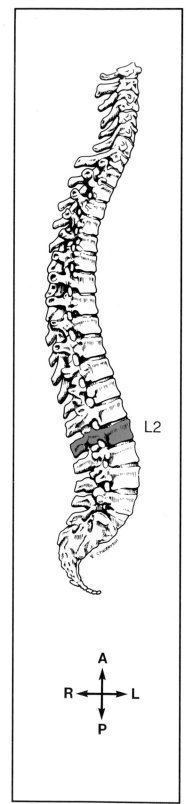

L2

A
R ← → L
P

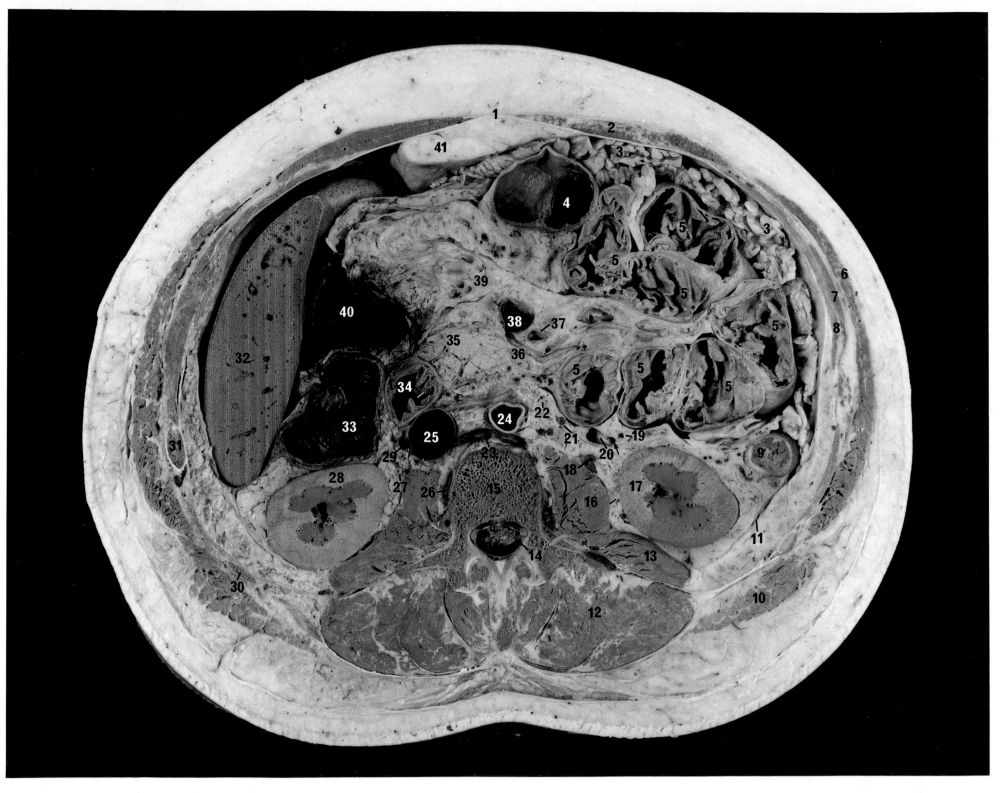

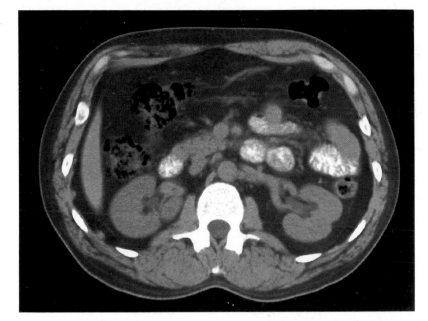

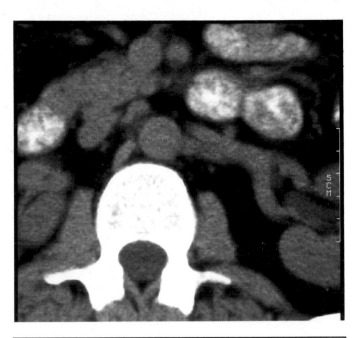

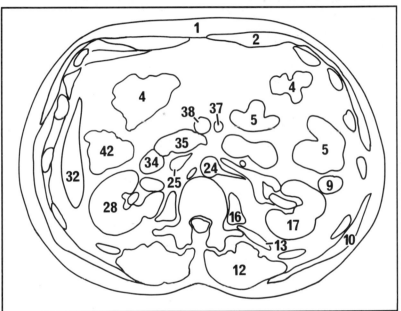

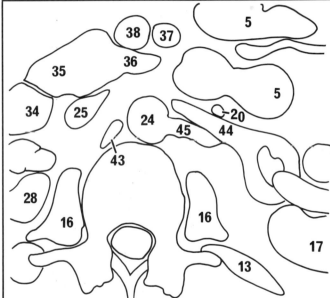

NOTES

This section passes through the body of the second lumbar vertebra (15).

The plane of section passes through a prominent left lumbar vein (23) as it passes posterior to the aorta (24) to drain into the inferior vena cava (25). Occasionally it may constitute the principal venous return from the left kidney, when it is termed a retroaortic renal vein.

The right testicular vein (29) drains directly into the inferior vena cava, whereas the left testicular vein (21) (together with the left suprarenal vein) drains into the left renal vein.

This section passes through the second part of the duodenum (34). The orifice of the ampulla of Vater on its papilla is marked with a white bristle.

On both the section and CT image the uncinate process of the pancreas (36) is clearly seen. This lies posterior to the superior mesenteric artery and vein (37, 38) and is closely related to the entry point of the left renal vein (44) into the inferior vena cava (25).

107

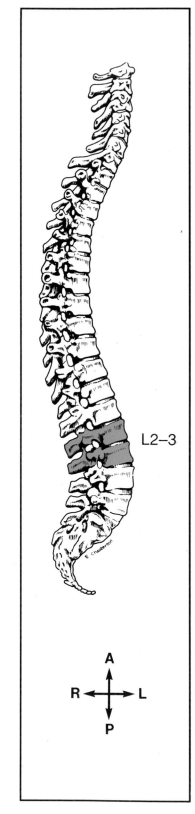

L2–3

A
R ←→ L
P

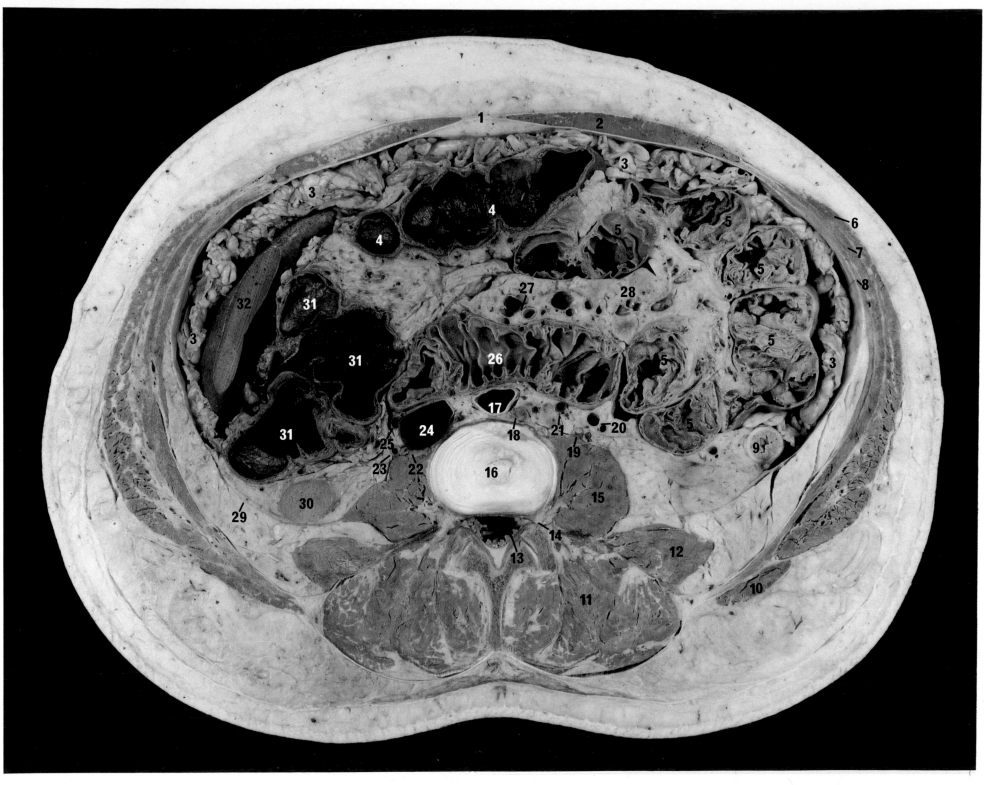

1 Linea alba
2 Rectus abdominis
3 Greater omentum
4 Transverse colon
5 Jejunum
6 External oblique
7 Internal oblique
8 Transversus abdominis
9 Descending colon
10 Latissimus dorsi
11 Erector spinae
12 Quadratus lumborum
13 Cauda equina within dural sheath
14 Root of second lumbar nerve
15 Psoas major
16 Intervertebral disc between the second and third lumbar vertebrae
17 Aorta
18 Para-aortic lymph node
19 Left ureter
20 Inferior mesenteric vein
21 Left testicular artery and vein
22 Right sympathetic chain
23 Right ureter
24 Inferior vena cava
25 Right testicular vein
26 Duodenum third part
27 Superior mesenteric artery and vein
28 Mesentery with mesenteric vessels
29 Renal fascia
30 Right kidney lower pole
31 Ascending colon and right colic (hepatic) flexure
32 Right lobe of liver

33 Ascending colon
34 Left kidney
35 Ileum

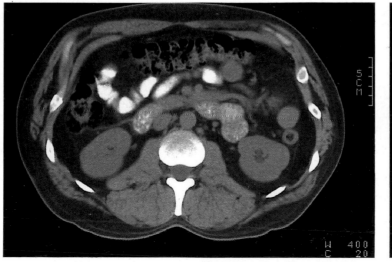
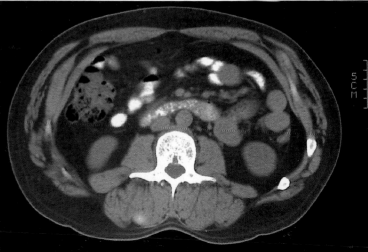
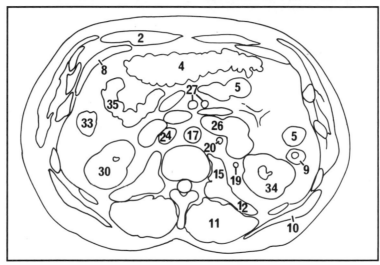
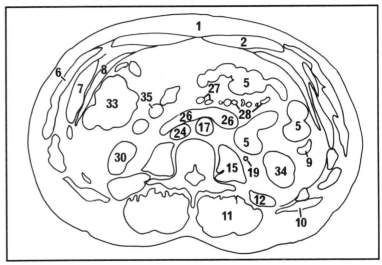

NOTES

This section passes through the intervertebral disc between the second and third lumbar vertebrae (16). It transects the most caudal part of the right lobe of the liver (32). The caudal extent of this lobe is variable and may project downwards in some subjects for a considerable distance as a broad tongue-like process (Riedel's lobe).

Note the third part of the duodenum (26) lying in the inverted V between the aorta (17) and the superior mesenteric vessels (27). Occasionally this produces obstruction of the third part of the duodenum (duodenal ileus).

Well seen in this section are the three layers of muscles which constitute the lateral part of the anterior abdominal wall; the external oblique (6), internal oblique (7) and transversus abdominis (8). Medially, their aponeuroses form the sheath which surrounds the rectus abdominis (2). The anterior sheath comprises the aponeurosis of the external oblique together with the split anterior portion of the internal oblique; the posterior sheath is made up of the aponeurosis of the transversus abdominis reinforced by the posterior portion of the internal oblique. Below a line roughly half-way between the umbilicus and the pubis the posterior sheath is deficient and all three aponeuroses pass in front of rectus to form the anterior sheath. These muscles are well demonstrated on CT image, section 47.

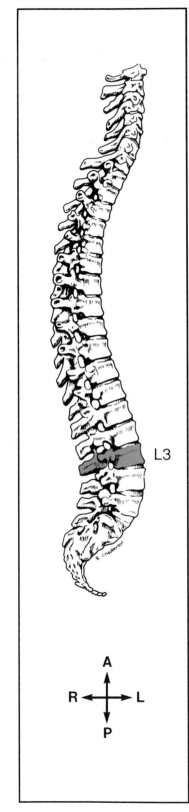

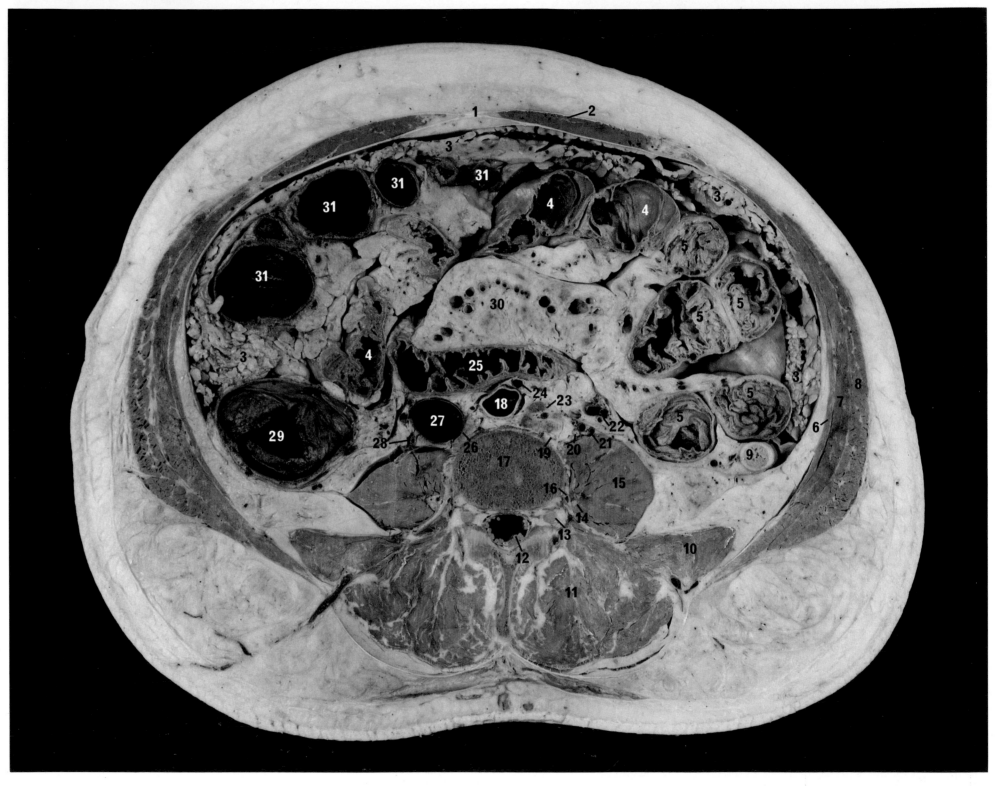

1 Linea alba
2 Rectus abdominis
3 Greater omentum
4 Ileum
5 Jejunum
6 Transversus abdominis
7 Internal oblique
8 External oblique
9 Descending colon
10 Quadratus lumborum
11 Erector spinae
12 Cauda equina within dural sheath
13 Dorsal root ganglion of third lumbar nerve
14 Ventral ramus of second lumbar nerve
15 Psoas major
16 Third lumbar artery
17 Body of third lumbar vertebra
18 Aorta
19 Left sympathetic chain
20 Left ureter
21 Left testicular artery and vein
22 Left colic artery and inferior mesenteric vein
23 Para-aortic lymph node
24 Inferior mesenteric artery
25 Duodenum third part
26 Right sympathetic chain
27 Inferior vena cava
28 Right ureter
29 Ascending colon
30 Mesentery with mesenteric vessels
31 Transverse colon

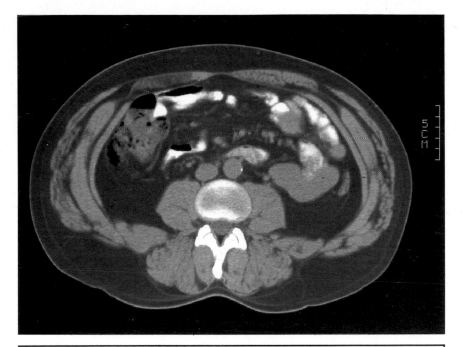

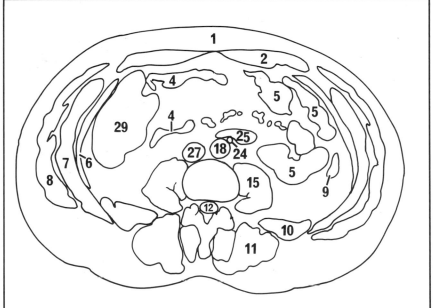

NOTES

This section passes through the body of the third lumbar vertebra (17). This is just distal to the origin of the inferior mesenteric artery (24) from the anterior aspect of the aorta (18) posterior to the third part of the duodenum (25). This section is now caudal to the liver and the kidneys.

The ventral ramus of the second lumbar nerve (14) is seen in this section as it passes downwards and laterally into the psoas major (15). The first three lumbar nerves and the greater part of the fourth form the lumbar plexus within the posterior part of the psoas major in front of the transverse processes of the lumbar vertebra.

Note the marked disparity between the patulous ascending colon (29) and the thick-walled narrow descending colon (9).

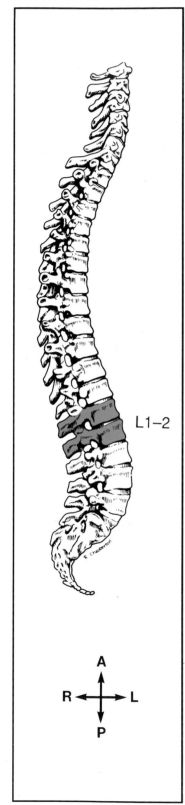

L1–2

A
R ← → L
P

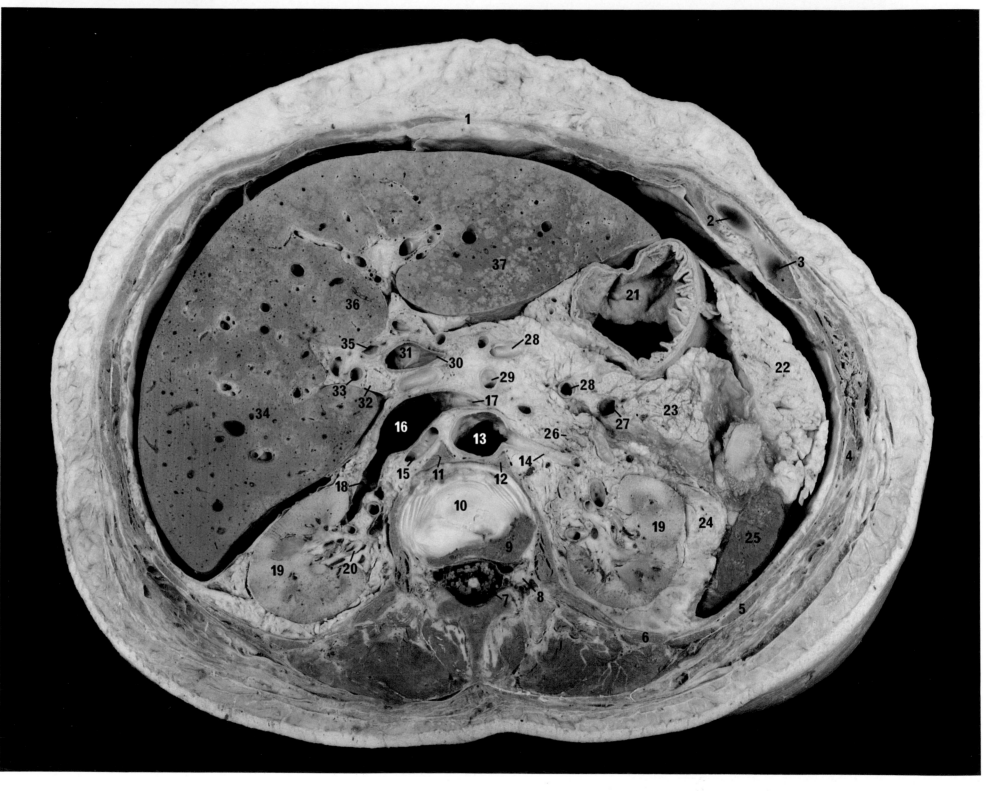

1 Linea alba
2 Eighth costal cartilage
3 Ninth rib/costal cartilage junction
4 Tenth rib
5 Eleventh rib
6 Twelfth rib
7 Cauda equina and termination of spinal cord within dural sheath
8 Dorsal root ganglion of first lumbar nerve
9 Part of body of first lumbar vertebra
10 Part of intervertebral disc between the first and second lumbar vertebrae
11 Right crus of diaphragm
12 Left crus of diaphragm
13 Aorta
14 Left renal artery
15 Right renal artery
16 Inferior vena cava
17 Left renal vein
18 Right renal vein
19 Kidney
20 Right ureter
21 Body of stomach
22 Greater omentum
23 Tail of pancreas
24 Perirenal fat within renal fascia
25 Spleen
26 Left suprarenal gland
27 Splenic vein
28 Splenic artery
29 Superior mesenteric artery
30 Termination of splenic vein
31 Commencement of portal vein
32 Lymph node in porta hepatis
33 Hepatic artery
34 Right lobe of liver
35 Common bile duct
36 Quadrate lobe of medial segment of left lobe of liver
37 Left lobe of liver, lateral segment

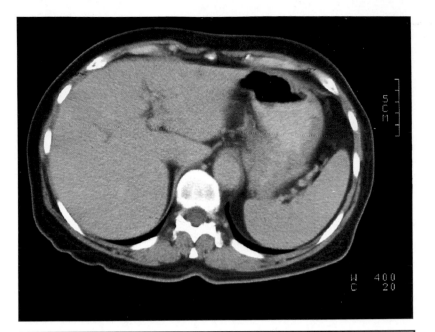

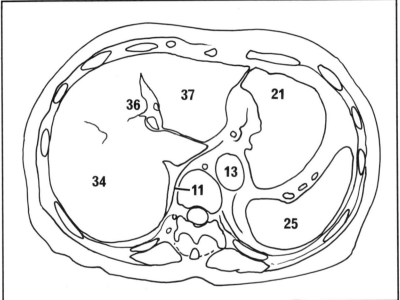

The sections through the female abdomen (48 and 49) should be compared with the male abdominal sections. There are, of course, wide individual variations in both the sexes, but a comparison of the male and female 'typical' abdomen reveals a greater accumulation of subcutaneous fat in the female in contrast to a higher proportion of intraperitoneal fat in the male subject.

This section passes through the intervertebral disc between the first and second lumbar vertebra.

This section shows well the quadrate lobe of the liver (36).

Although the common bile duct (35) is usually the most anterolateral structure in the free (right) edge of the lesser omentum, variations are common. In this elderly female, the hepatic artery (33) is tortuous and thus is unusually lateral. Anomalies of the hepatic artery are common. In 12% of cases the right hepatic artery or an accessory right hepatic artery derives from the superior mesenteric artery. The left hepatic artery or an accessory hepatic artery may originate from the left gastric, splenic or superior mesenteric artery. Occasionally one or other of these vessels derives directly from the aorta.

Note the caudal tip of the left suprarenal gland (26), which may extend down to the left renal vein.

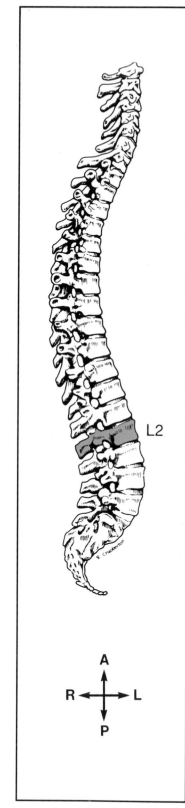

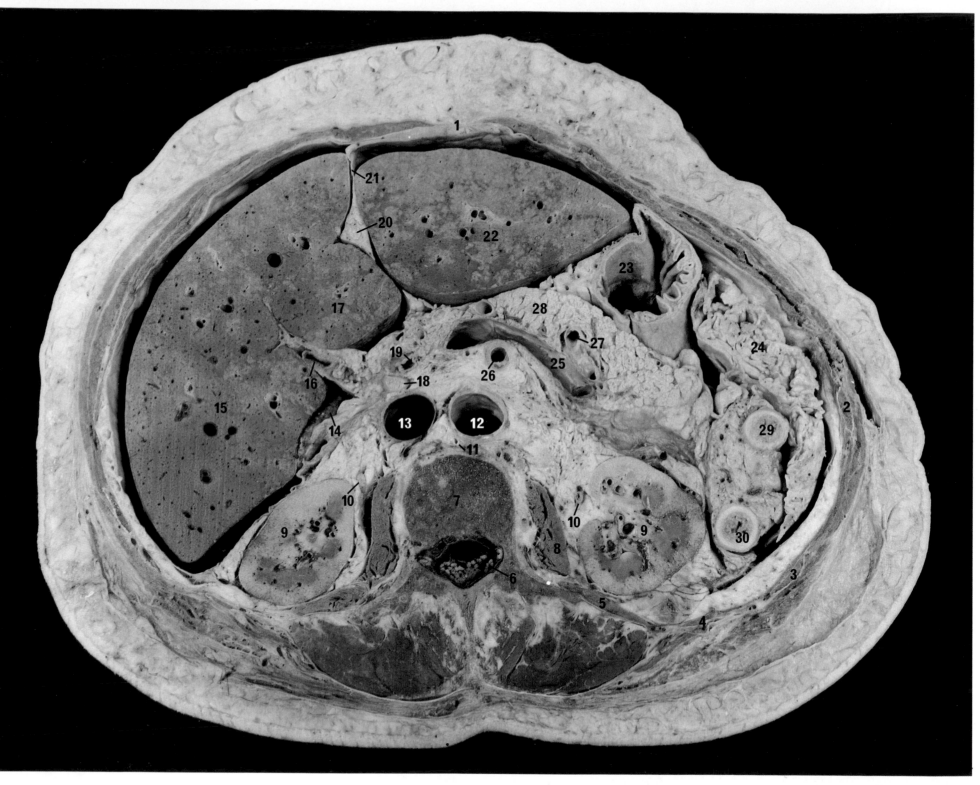

1 Linea alba
2 Tenth rib
3 Eleventh rib
4 Twelfth rib
5 Quadratus lumborum
6 Cauda equina within dural sheath
7 Body of second lumbar vertebra
8 Psoas major
9 Kidney
10 Ureter
11 Cisterna chyli
12 Aorta
13 Inferior vena cava
14 Caudate lobe of liver
15 Right lobe of liver
16 Neck of gall bladder
17 Left lobe of liver (medial segment)
18 Lymph node in porta hepatis
19 Common bile duct
20 Ligamentum teres
21 Falciform ligament
22 Left lobe of liver (lateral segment)
23 Body of stomach
24 Greater omentum
25 Splenic vein
26 Superior mesenteric artery
27 Splenic artery
28 Body of pancreas
29 Transverse colon
30 Descending colon

31 Spleen
32 Right suprarenal gland

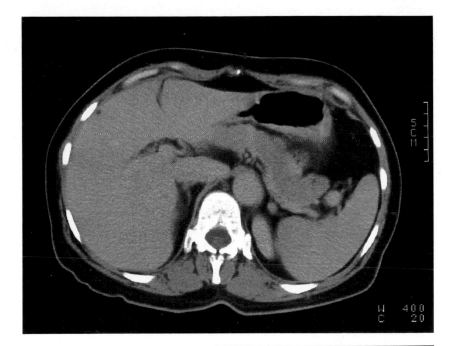

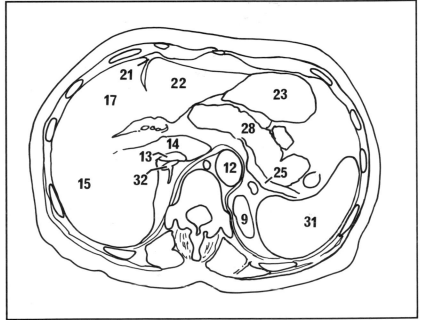

NOTES

This section lies just caudal to the left colic (splenic) flexure which joins the transverse colon (29) to the descending colon (30).

The tip of the papillary process of the caudate lobe of the liver (14) can be seen as a separate structure in the gap medial to the right lobe of the liver. The ligamentum teres (20) is the fibrotic remnant of the obliterated left umbilical vein. The falciform ligament divides the *morphological* left lobe of the liver into a lateral segment (22) and medial segment (17). The visceral aspect of this, between the falciform ligament and the gall bladder bed (16) forms the *anatomical* quadrate lobe.

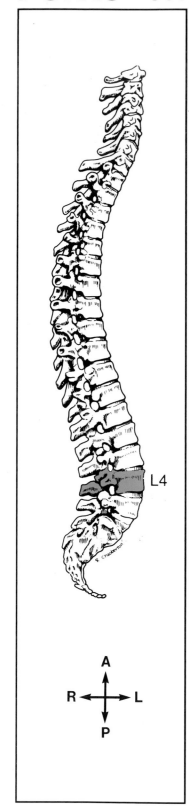

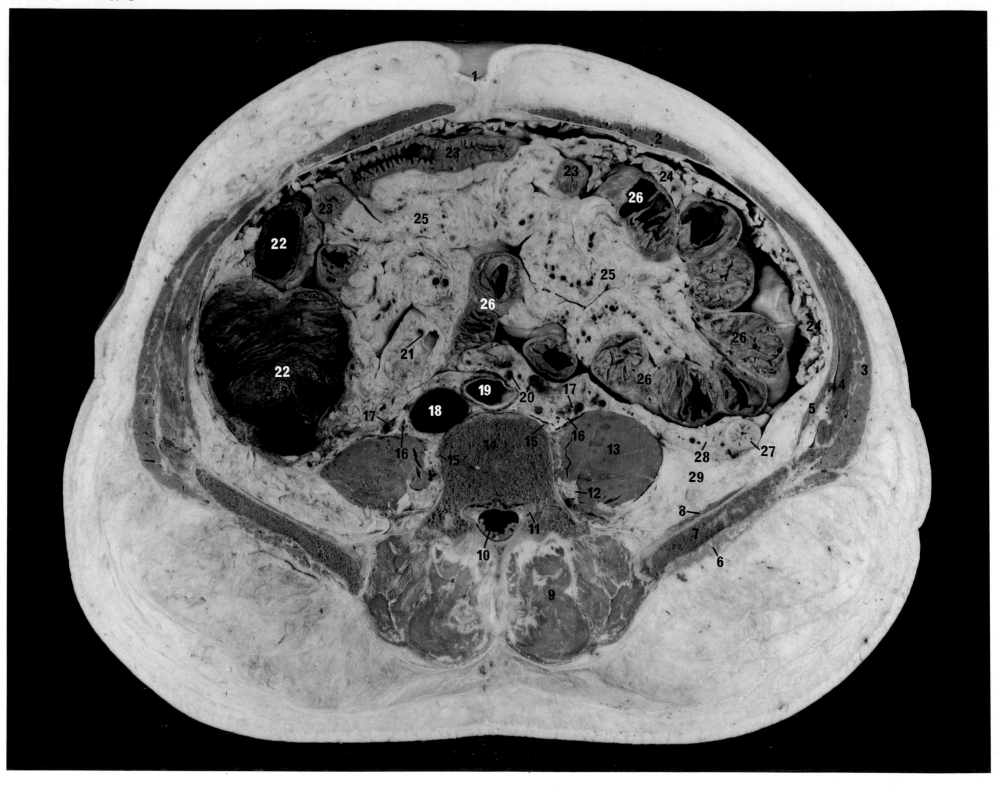

1 Umbilicus
2 Rectus abdominis
3 External oblique
4 Internal oblique
5 Transversus abdominis
6 Gluteus medius
7 Ilium
8 Iliacus
9 Erector spinae
10 Cauda equina within dural sheath
11 Dorsal root ganglion of fourth lumbar nerve
12 Ventral ramus of third lumbar nerve
13 Psoas major
14 Body of fourth lumbar vertebra
15 Lumbar sympathetic chain
16 Ureter
17 Testicular artery and vein
18 Inferior vena cava
19 Aorta
20 Inferior mesenteric artery and vein
21 Right colic artery and vein
22 Ascending colon
23 Jejunum
24 Greater omentum
25 Mesentery of small intestine
26 Ileum
27 Descending colon
28 Anterior pararenal fat of retroperitoneum
29 Posterior pararenal fat of retroperitoneum

30 Appendix vermiformis

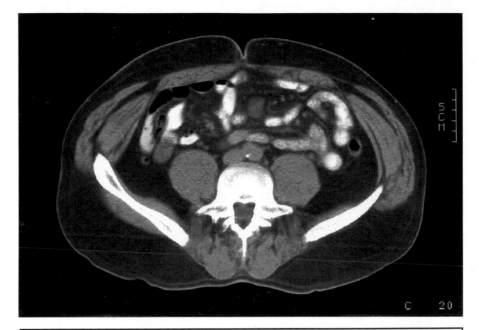

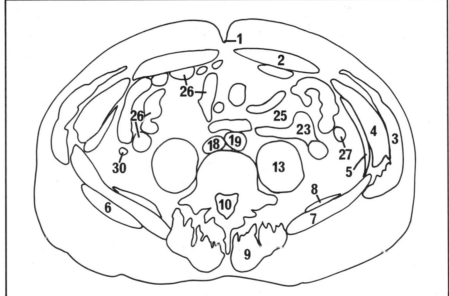

NOTES

This section passes through the body of the fourth lumbar vertebra (14), the cranial portion of the iliac crests (7) and the umbilicus (1). There are quite wide individual variations in these landmarks; however the umbilicus is usually at the L3/4 intervertebral disc level and the iliac crest at the level of L4.

The inferior mesenteric artery (20) has just arisen from the aorta at the level of the third lumbar vertebra. More caudally, it will give rise to the superior rectal artery (see section 51). The accompanying inferior mesenteric vein (20) has a long ascending retroperitoneal course to enter the splenic vein.

The aorta (19) is commencing to bifurcate on both the section and the CT image.

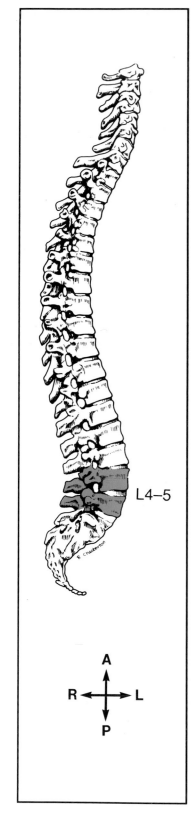

L4–5

A
R ← → L
P

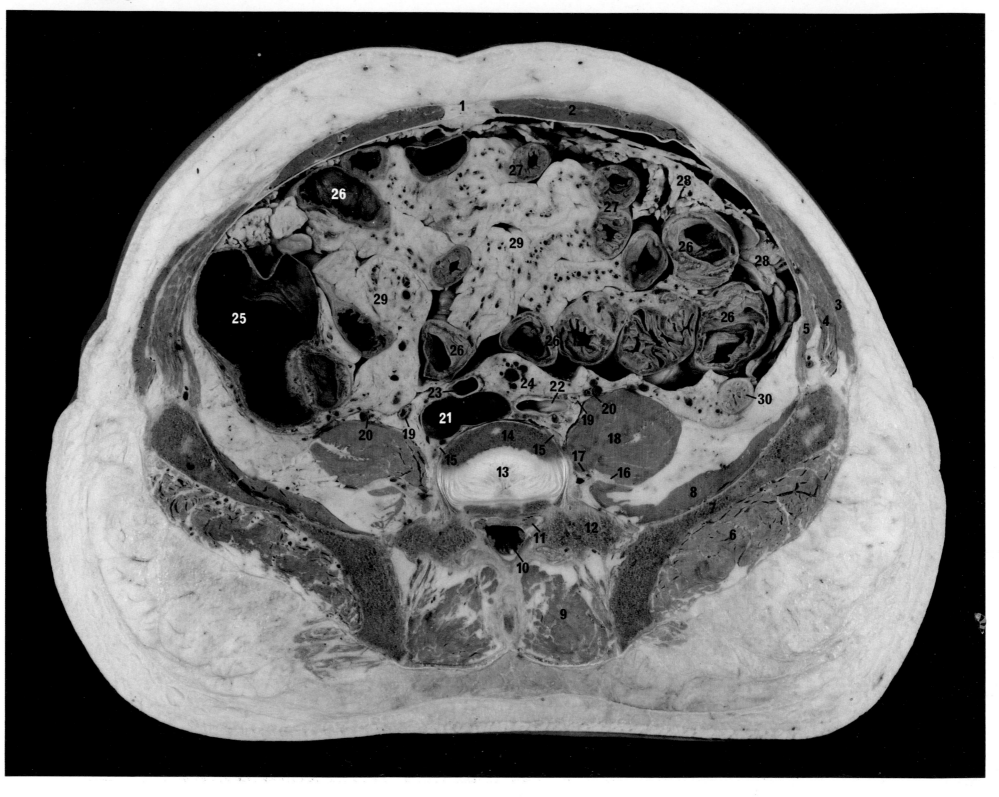

1 Linea alba
2 Rectus abdominis
3 External oblique
4 Internal oblique
5 Transversus abdominis
6 Gluteus medius
7 Ilium
8 Iliacus
9 Erector spinae
10 Cauda equina within dural sheath
11 Root of fifth lumbar nerve
12 Transverse process of fifth lumbar vertebra
13 Part of intervertebral disc between the fourth and fifth lumbar vertebrae
14 Part of body of fourth lumbar vertebra
15 Lumbar sympathetic chain
16 Femoral nerve
17 Obturator nerve
18 Psoas major
19 Ureter
20 Testicular artery and vein
21 Inferior vena cava at origin
22 Left common iliac artery
23 Right common iliac artery
24 Superior rectal artery and vein
25 Ascending colon
26 Ileum
27 Jejunum
28 Greater omentum
29 Mesentery of small bowel
30 Descending colon

31 Appendix vermiformis

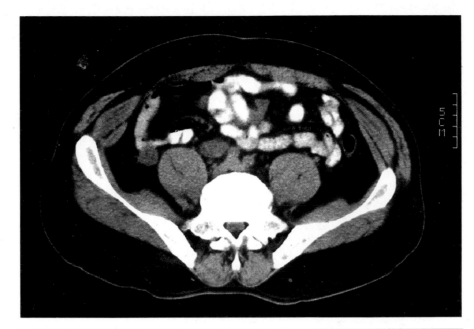

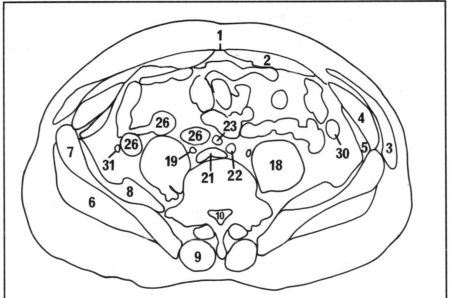

NOTES

This section transects the intervertebral disc between the fourth and fifth lumbar vertebrae (13).

The lumbar sympathetic chain (15) is well visualized as it lies on the fourth lumbar vertebral body (14); it is overlapped on the right by the inferior vena cava (21) and by the common iliac artery on the left (22). More cranially it lies just lateral to the aorta, as can be seen in section 50.

The transverse processes of the fifth lumbar vertebra (12) are bulky and all but reach the sacrum, particularly (in this specimen) on the left side. Reference to section 52 shows that there is partial sacralization of L5, a very common variation.

The superior rectal artery (24) is the continuation of the inferior mesenteric artery after this has given off its left colic branch (see section 50).

The inferior vena cava (21) is seen at its commencement, and its oval shape in the section (more markedly oval in the CT image) is produced by the convergence of the two common iliac veins at this level.

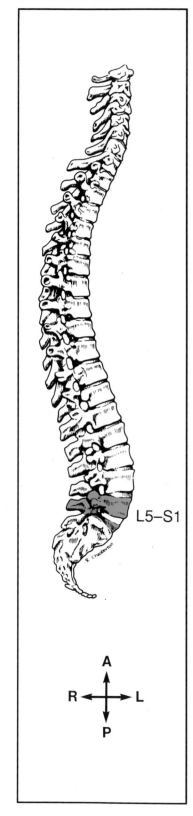

L5–S1

A
R ← → L
P

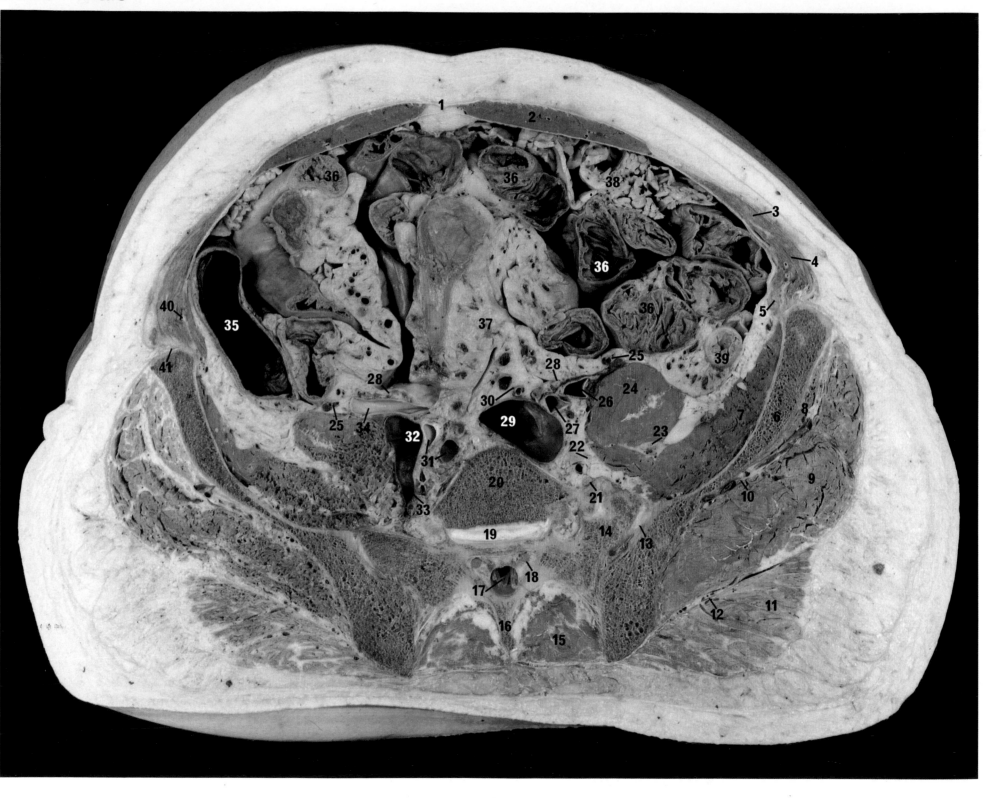

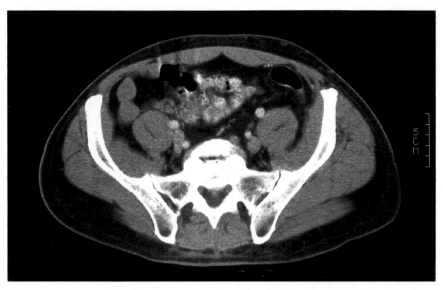

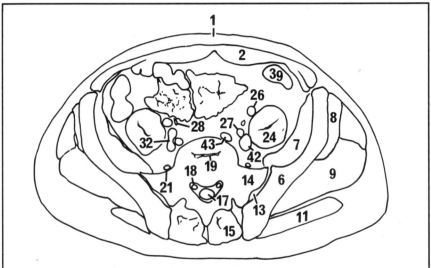

NOTES

This section traverses the sacro-iliac joint (13), the lumbosacral disc (19) and the lower part of the body of the fifth lumbar vertebra (20). There is some asymmetry of the lateral mass of the sacrum (14) in this subject, the left side being larger. This is because there is a small articulation (which is just visible) between the left sacral mass and the 'sacralized' left L5 transverse process (see also section 51). These variations are very common.

An intravenous injection of contrast medium was given before the CT image series, hence the opacification of the blood vessels.

The superior gluteal vessels (31) arise from the internal iliac vessels. Together with the superior gluteal nerve (10), they emerge from the pelvis through the greater sciatic foramen *above* piriformis, then run between and supply gluteus medius (9) and gluteus minimus (8). The inferior gluteal artery, vein and nerve (12) emerge *below* piriformis and supply gluteus maximus (11).

121

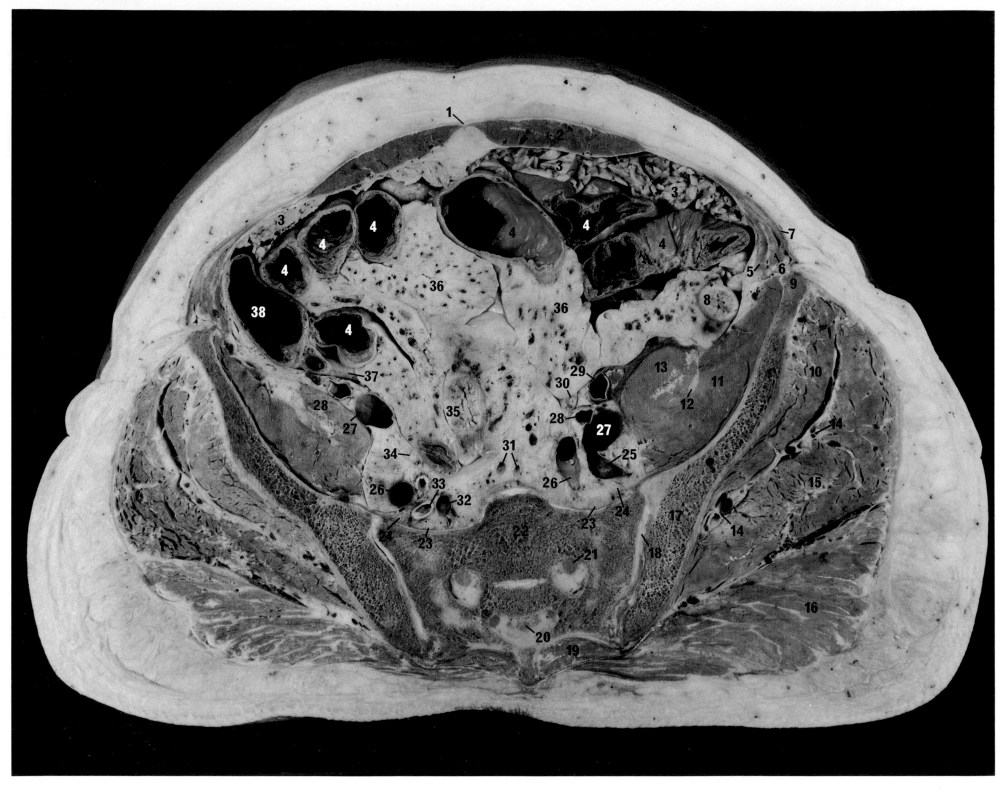

1 Linea alba
2 Rectus abdominis
3 Greater omentum
4 Ileum
5 Transversus abdominis
6 Internal oblique
7 External oblique aponeurosis
8 Descending colon
9 Anterior superior iliac spine
10 Gluteus minimus
11 Iliacus
12 Femoral nerve
13 Psoas major
14 Superior gluteal artery and vein
15 Gluteus medius
16 Gluteus maximus
17 Ilium
18 Sacro-iliac joint
19 Erector spinae
20 Filum terminale within sacral canal
21 Second sacral nerve root
22 Sacrum second segment
23 Lumbosacral trunk
24 Obturator nerve
25 Iliolumbar vein
26 Internal iliac vein
27 External iliac vein
28 Internal iliac artery
29 External iliac artery
30 Left ureter
31 Median sacral artery and vein
32 Superior gluteal vein
33 Superior gluteal artery
34 Right ureter
35 Sigmoid colon
36 Mesentery of ileum
37 Appendix vermiformis
38 Caecum

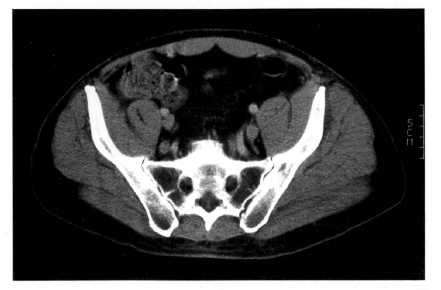

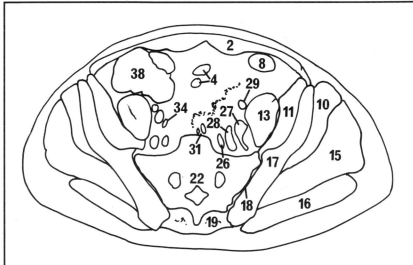

NOTES

This section transects the second segment of the sacrum (22). Note that in this subject the gluteal muscles on the right side are smaller and paler than on the left (10, 15, 16). This subject had suffered a cerebrovascular accident which resulted in a right-sided paresis.

The appendix vermiformis (37) lies posterior to the ileum (4) in this section – the retro-ileal position. Much more commonly the appendix lies behind the caecum (in about 65% of cases) or descends into the pelvis (30% of cases) (see CT images, sections 50 and 51).

The superior gluteal vessels in their pelvic (32, 33) and gluteal (14) course are again well demonstrated (see section 52).

S3

A
R ← → L
P

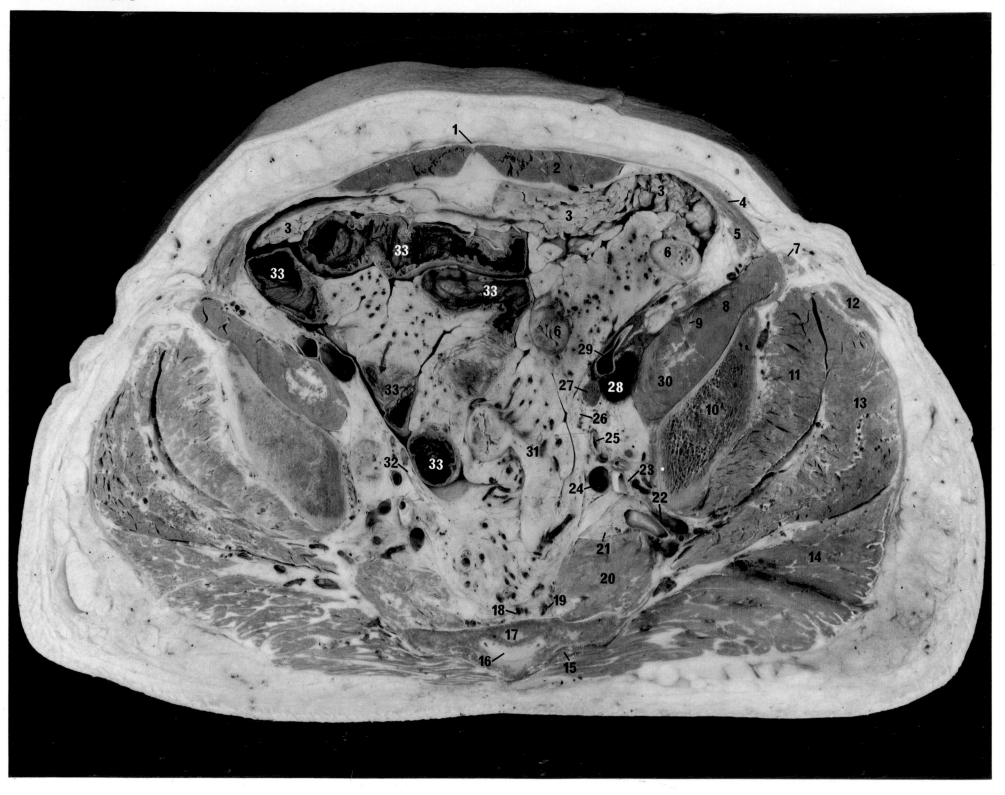

1 Linea alba
2 Rectus abdominis
3 Greater omentum
4 Internal oblique
5 Transversus abdominis
6 Sigmoid colon
7 Sartorius
8 Iliacus
9 Femoral nerve
10 Ilium
11 Gluteus minimus
12 Tensor fasciae latae
13 Gluteus medius
14 Gluteus maximus
15 Erector spinae
16 Sacral canal
17 Sacrum third segment
18 Median sacral artery and vein
19 Lateral sacral artery and vein
20 Piriformis
21 Sciatic nerve
22 Superior gluteal artery and vein
23 Obturator artery and vein
24 Internal iliac vein
25 Internal iliac artery
26 Left ureter
27 Lymph node
28 External iliac vein
29 External iliac artery
30 Psoas major
31 Sigmoid mesocolon
32 Right ureter
33 Ileum

34 Bladder
35 Vas deferens
36 Inferior epigastric artery

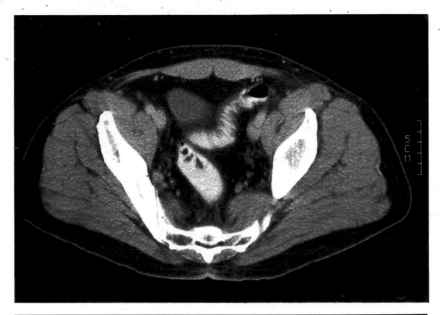

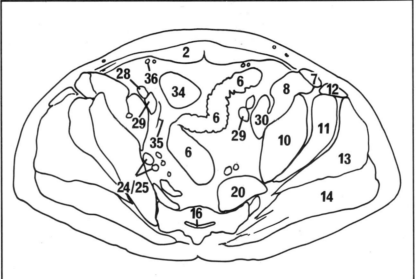

NOTES

This section passes through the sacrum at its third segment (17).

Piriformis (20) arises from the front of the sacrum by three digitations, attached to the portions of bone between the pelvic sacral foramina and also to the grooves leading laterally from these foramina. The superior gluteal vessels (22), together with the superior gluteal nerve, pass above piriformis through the greater sciatic foramen. In this subject, piriformis is paler and less bulky on the right side than on the left as a result of a previous cerebrovascular accident (see section 53). Piriformis is a bulky muscle which must be traversed when using the greater sciatic foramen as a route for percutaneous pelvic aspiration. On the CT image there is asymmetry of the piriformis muscles due to a degree of scoliosis.

The ureter (26) descends into the pelvis characteristically immediately anterior to the internal iliac artery (25). It lies immediately deep to the pelvic peritoneum, crossed only by the vas deferens, which is seen in section 55.

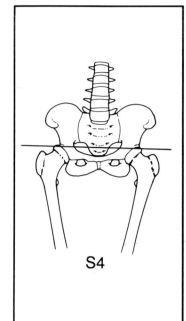

S4

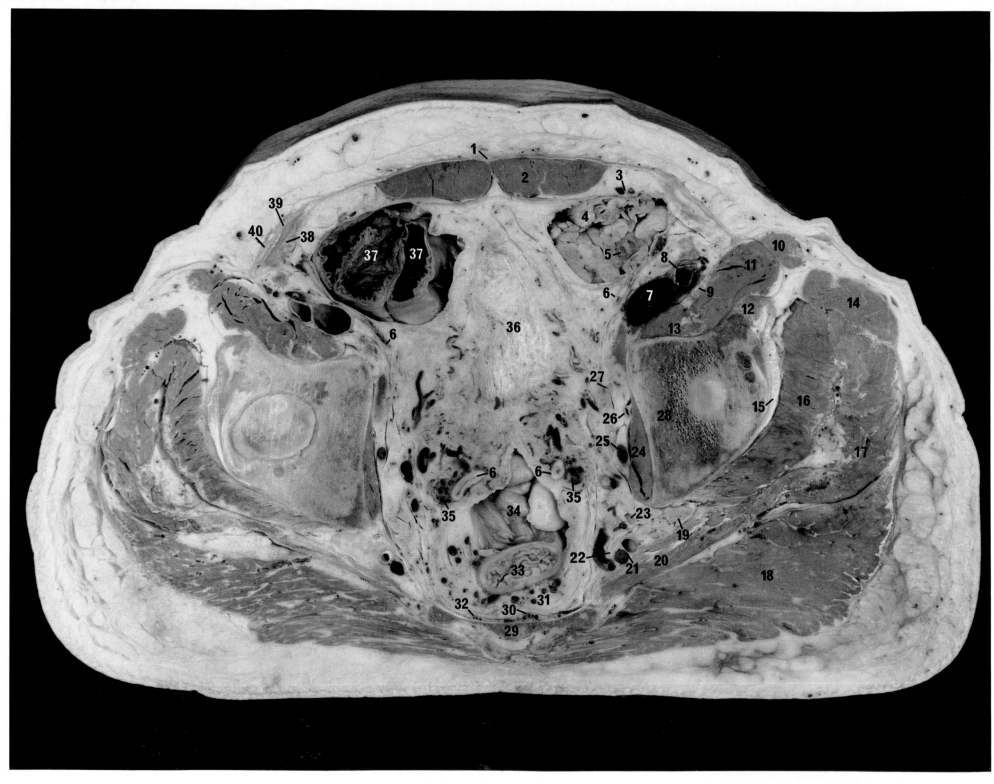

A
R ← → L
P

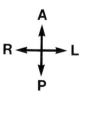

1 Linea alba	24 Obturator internus
2 Rectus abdominis	25 Obturator vein
3 Inferior epigastric artery and vein	26 Obturator artery
	27 Obturator nerve
4 Greater omentum	28 Acetabulum (ilial portion)
5 Sigmoid colon	29 Sacrum fourth segment
6 Vas deferens	30 Median sacral artery and vein
7 External iliac vein	
8 External iliac artery	31 Superior rectal artery and vein
9 Femoral nerve	
10 Sartorius	32 Lateral sacral artery and vein
11 Iliacus	
12 Rectus femoris straight head tendon	33 Rectum
	34 Rectosigmoid junction
13 Psoas major and tendon	35 Seminal vesicle
14 Tensor fasciae latae	36 Fundus of bladder
15 Iliofemoral ligament	37 Ileum
16 Gluteus minimus	38 Transversus abdominis
17 Gluteus medius	39 Internal oblique
18 Gluteus maximus	40 External oblique
19 Sciatic nerve	
20 Piriformis	41 Perirectal fat
21 Inferior gluteal artery and vein	42 Pararectal fat (with branches of internal iliac artery and vein)
22 Pudendal nerve	
23 Internal pudendal artery	43 Perirectal fascia

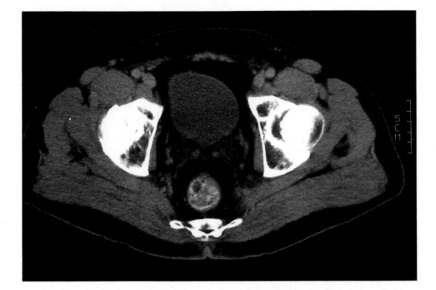

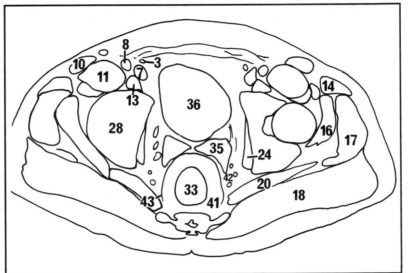

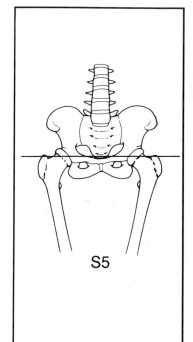

S5

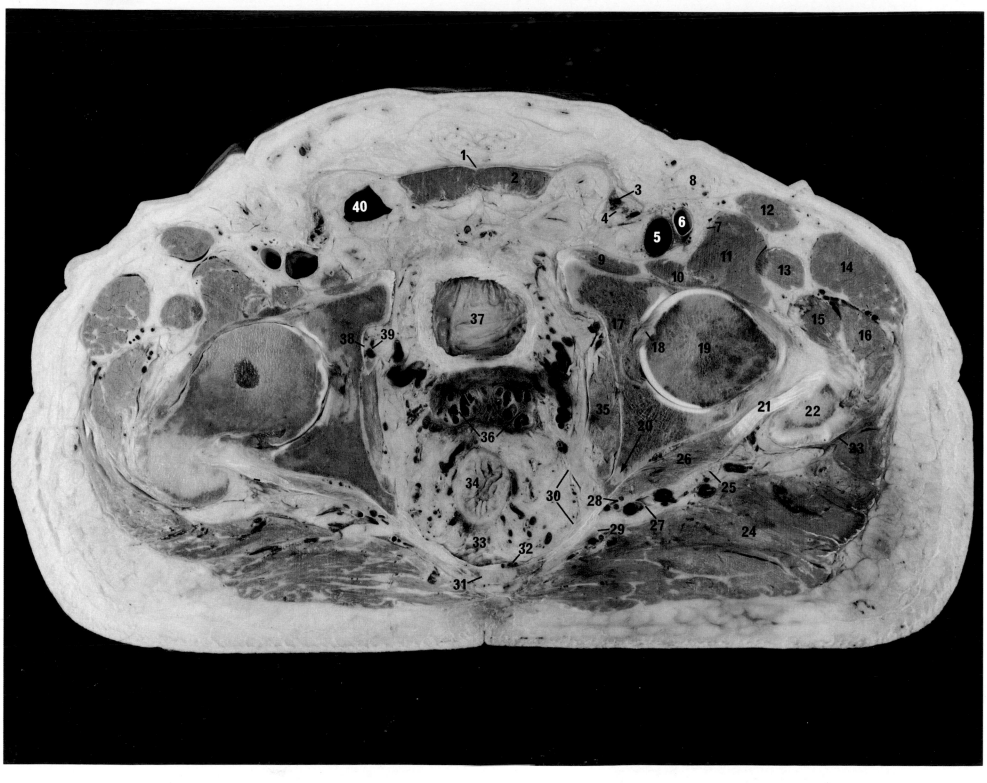

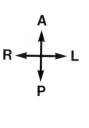

A
R ← → L
P

1 Linea alba
2 Rectus abdominis
3 Spermatic cord
4 Vas deferens
5 Femoral vein
6 Femoral artery
7 Femoral nerve
8 Lymph node
9 Pectineus
10 Psoas major and tendon
11 Iliacus
12 Sartorius
13 Rectus femoris
14 Tensor fasciae latae
15 Gluteus minimus
16 Gluteus medius
17 Acetabulum (pubic portion)
18 Ligamentum teres
19 Femoral head
20 Ischium leading to ischial spine (arrowed)
21 Obturator internus tendon
22 Greater trochanter
23 Trochanteric bursa
24 Gluteus maximus
25 Sciatic nerve
26 Gemellus superior
27 Inferior gluteal artery and vein
28 Pudendal nerve and internal pudendal artery and vein
29 Sacrospinous ligament
30 Perirectal fascia separating perirectal fat from pararectal fat
31 Sacrum fifth segment
32 Lateral sacral artery and vein
33 Superior rectal artery and vein in perirectal fat
34 Rectum
35 Obturator internus
36 Seminal vesicle
37 Bladder
38 Obturator nerve
39 Obturator artery and vein
40 Patent processus vaginalis (indirect inguinal hernia sac)

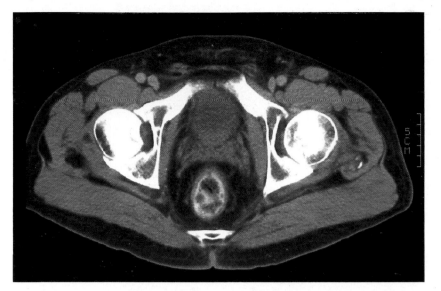

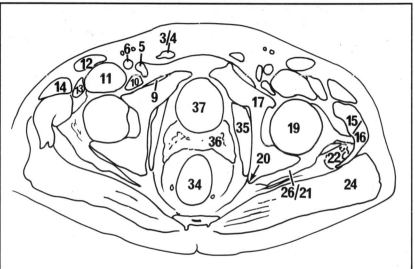

NOTES

This section traverses the last, fifth, segment of the sacrum (31). The sacrospinous ligament (29) is transected as it passes forward to the ischial spine (20).

This section gives an excellent illustration of the hip joint at the level of the ligamentum teres (18).

The superior rectal vessels (33) can be seen as they lie in the loose perirectal fat, which also contains lymphatic vessels, lymph nodes and the pelvic plexuses lying on the rectal wall. The perirectal fat is separated by the perirectal fascia (30) from the pararectal fat.

Note that this subject has an indirect inguinal hernia sac on the right side (40).

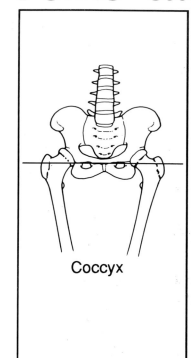

Coccyx

A
R ← → L
P

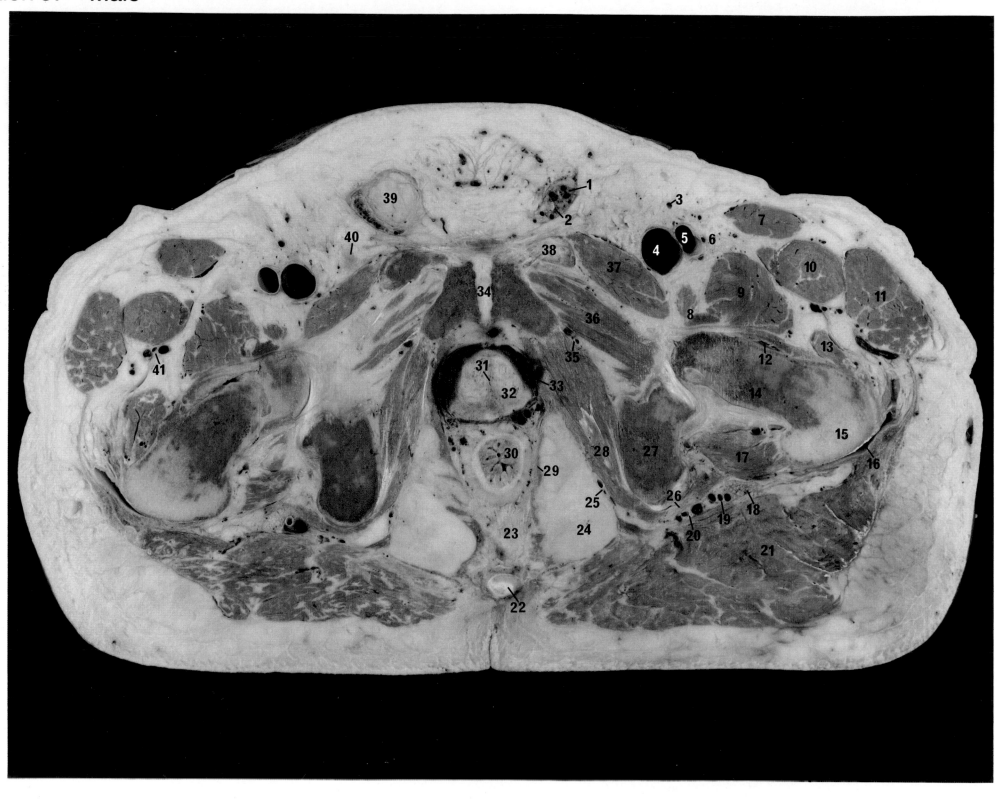

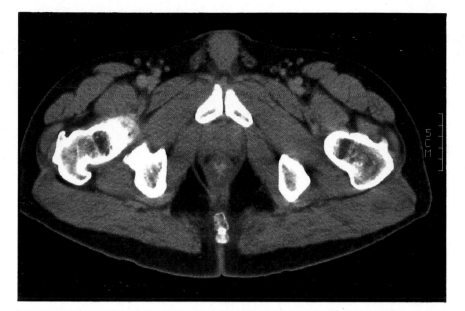

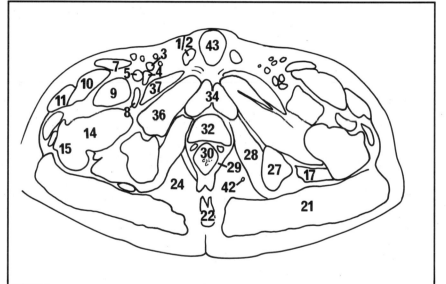

NOTES

This section passes through the coccyx (22) and the symphysis pubis (34). In the standing position, the horizontal plane which passes through the coccyx corresponds to the superior margin of the symphysis.

The ischiorectal fossa (24) is wedge-shaped with its base pointing to the surface of the perineum, while its apex is the junction of obturator internus (28) and levator ani (29) covered respectively by the obturator fascia and the inferior fascia of the pelvic diaphragm. Medially it is bounded by the external anal sphincter and levator ani, laterally by the tuberosity of the ischium and the obturator fascia and posteriorly by the lower border of gluteus maximus (21) and the sacrotuberous ligament. Anteriorly lies the urogenital diaphragm, but the fossa is prolonged as a narrow recess above this diaphragm, where it is limited by the fusion between the inferior fascia of the pelvic diaphragm and the superior fascia of the urogenital diaphragm.

The internal pudendal vessels and the pudendal nerve (20) enter the perineum through the lesser sciatic foramen and then traverse the pudendal canal of Alcock (25). This canal comprises a special sheath of fascia fused with the lower part of the obturator fascia.

The left common femoral artery (5) is about to divide into the superficial femoral and profunda femoris on the section: on the CT image this has already taken place.

The spermatic cord (1) and vas deferens (2) are clearly seen on the left side. On the right these are compressed by extraperitoneal fat related to this subject's indirect inguinal hernia (39). This hernia is clearly seen in section 56.

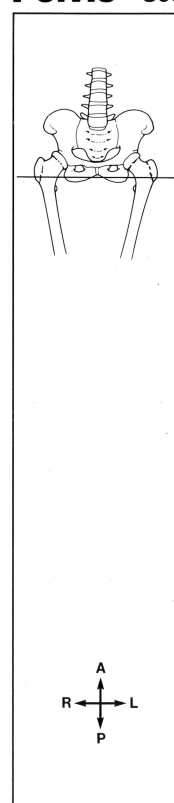

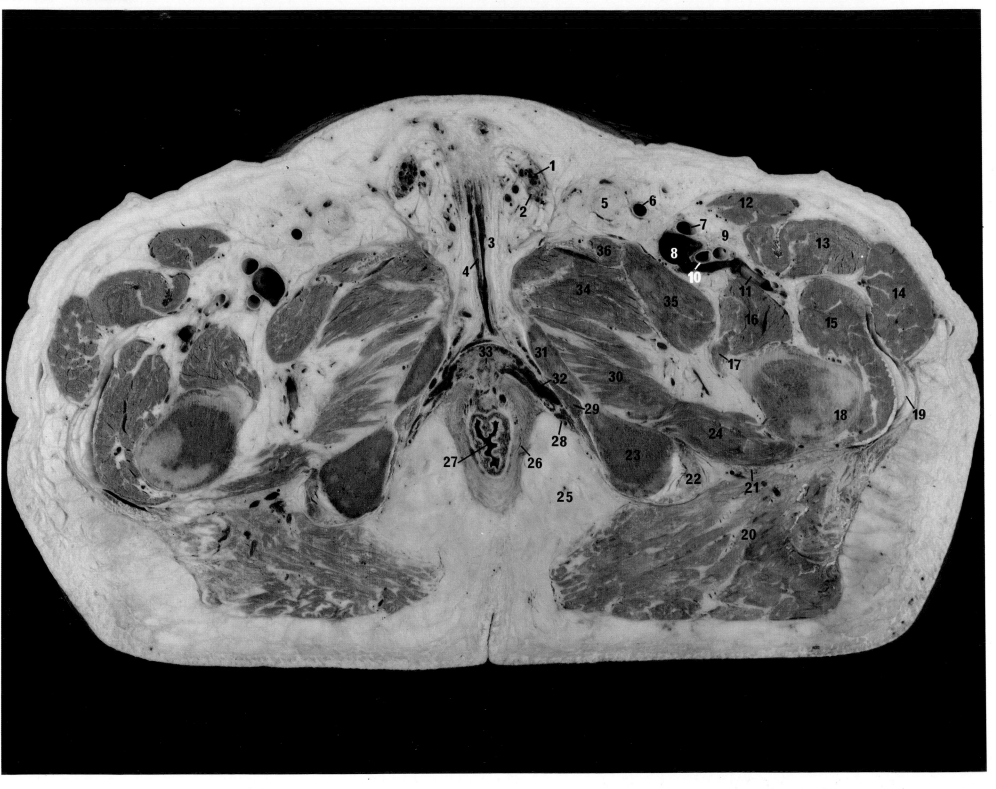

1 Spermatic cord
2 Vas deferens
3 Tunica albuginea of penis
4 Corpus cavernosum (body)
5 Inguinal lymph node
6 Great saphenous vein
7 Superficial femoral artery
8 Femoral vein
9 Femoral nerve
10 Profunda femoris artery
11 Lateral circumflex femoral vein
12 Sartorius
13 Rectus femoris
14 Tensor fasciae latae
15 Vastus lateralis
16 Iliacus
17 Tendon of psoas major
18 Greater trochanter
19 Trochanteric bursa
20 Gluteus maximus
21 Sciatic nerve
22 Biceps femoris tendon
23 Ischial tuberosity
24 Quadratus femoris
25 Ischiorectal fat
26 Levator ani
27 Anorectal junction
28 Pudendal canal
29 Obturator internus
30 Obturator externus
31 Pubis – inferior ramus
32 Corpus cavernosum (crus)
33 Urethra (in distal prostate)
34 Adductor brevis
35 Pectineus
36 Adductor longus

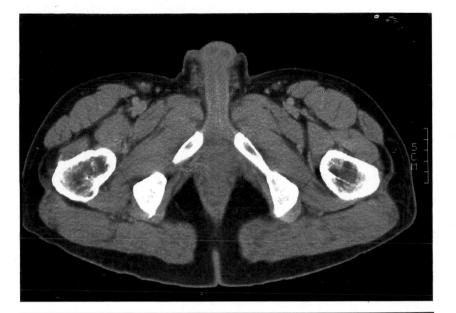

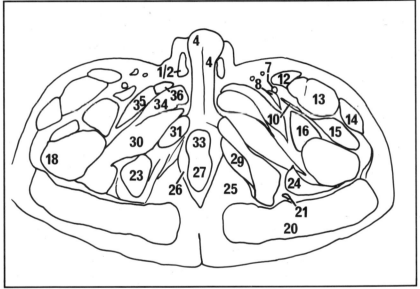

NOTES

This section lies caudal to the coccyx and pubis but passes through the level of the ischial tuberosity (23). The plane of section cuts through the anorectal junction (27), around which lies the levator ani (26).

The ischiorectal fossa, filled with fat (25), which is described in section 57, can be seen to communicate with the fossa on the other side posterior to the anal canal. The inferior rectal artery is clearly seen in the centre of the fossa on the left side.

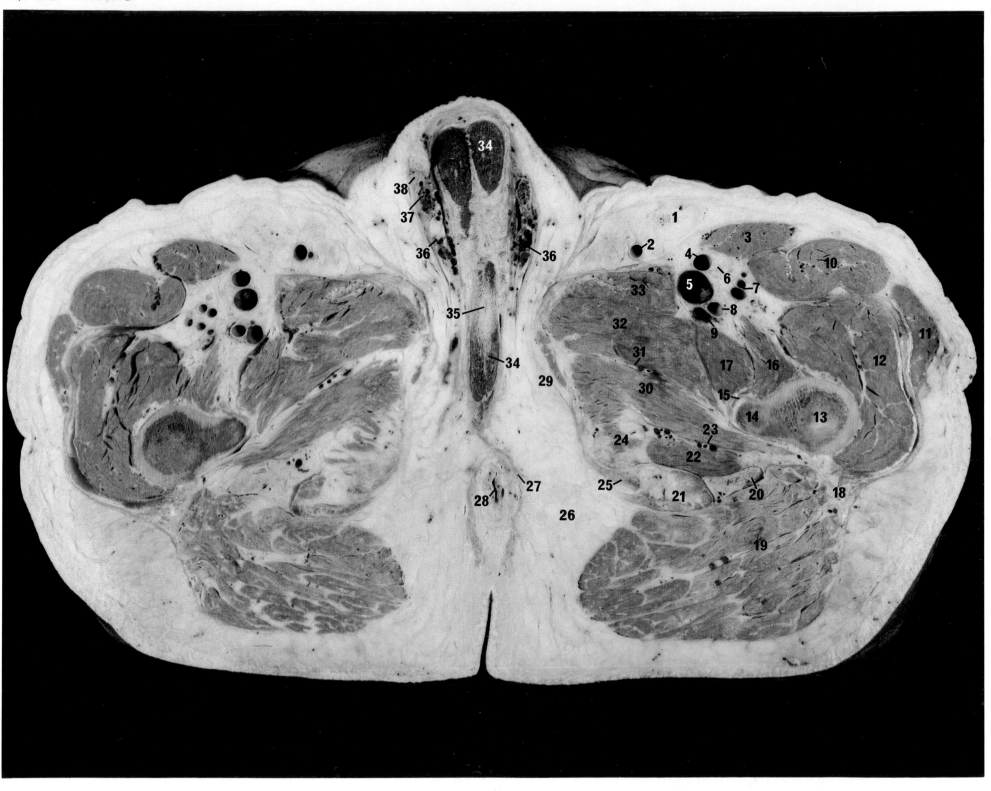

1 Inguinal lymph node
2 Great saphenous vein
3 Sartorius
4 Superficial femoral artery
5 Superficial femoral vein
6 Femoral nerve
7 Lateral circumflex femoral artery and vein
8 Profunda femoris artery
9 Profunda femoris vein
10 Rectus femoris
11 Tensor fasciae latae
12 Vastus lateralis
13 Femur
14 Lesser trochanter
15 Tendon of psoas major
16 Iliacus
17 Pectineus
18 Gluteus maximus tendon
19 Gluteus maximus
20 Sciatic nerve
21 Biceps femoris and semitendinosus tendons
22 Quadratus femoris
23 Profunda femoris artery and vein: first perforating branches
24 Semimembranosus
25 Ischium
26 Ischiorectal fat
27 Levator ani
28 Anal canal
29 Gracilis
30 Adductor magnus
31 Obturator nerve deep branch
32 Adductor brevis
33 Adductor longus
34 Corpus cavernosum
35 Urethra
36 Pampiniform plexus
37 Spermatic cord
38 Vas deferens

39 Corpus cavernosum (crus)
40 Obturator externus

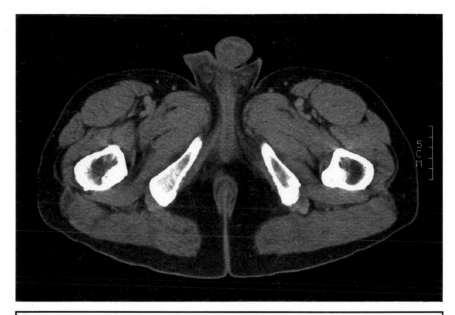

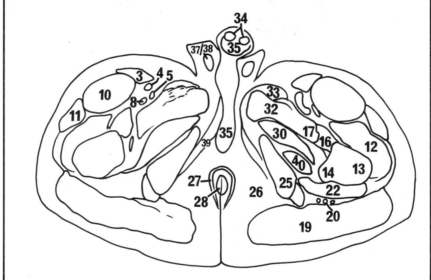

NOTES

This section is completely below the pelvic girdle and transects the upper ends of the femoral shafts (13) at the level of the lesser trochanter (14). It transects the anal canal (28).

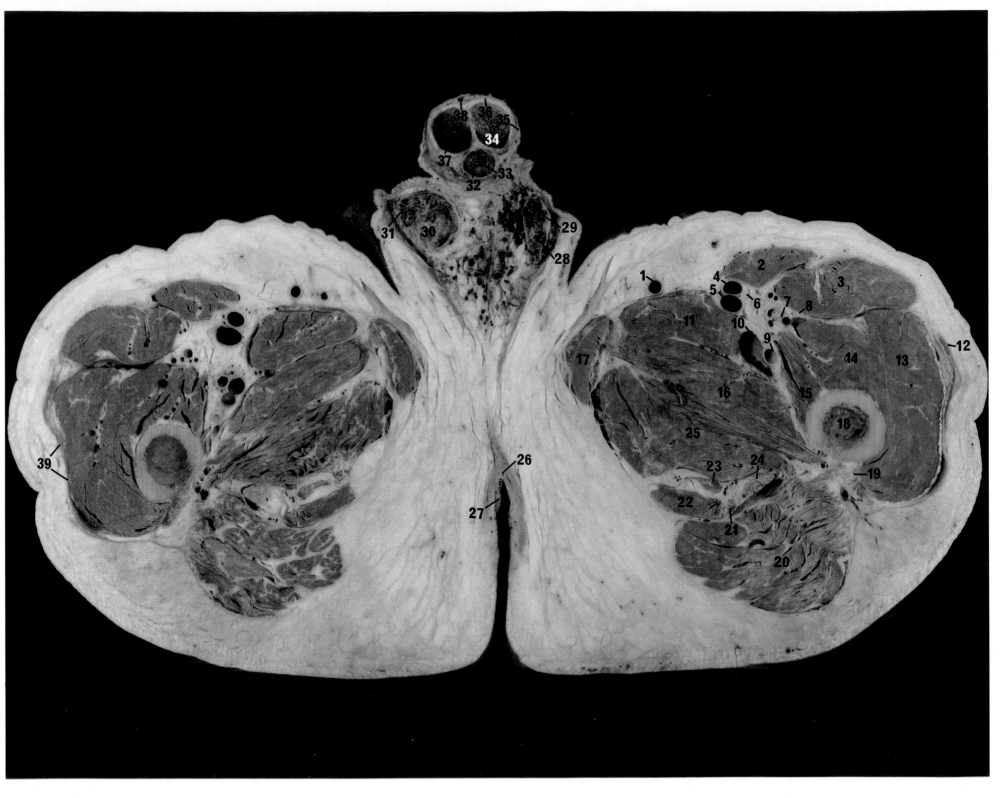

1 Great saphenous vein
2 Sartorius
3 Rectus femoris
4 Superficial femoral artery
5 Superficial femoral vein
6 Saphenous nerve
7 Lateral circumflex femoral artery and vein (inferior branch)
8 Femoral nerve (branch to quadriceps)
9 Profunda femoris artery
10 Profunda femoris vein
11 Adductor longus
12 Tensor fasciae latae
13 Vastus lateralis
14 Vastus intermedius
15 Vastus medialis
16 Adductor brevis
17 Gracilis
18 Femoral shaft
19 Gluteus maximus tendon
20 Gluteus maximus
21 Biceps femoris – tendon of long head
22 Semimembranosus
23 Semitendinosus tendon
24 Sciatic nerve
25 Adductor magnus
26 External anal sphincter
27 Anal verge
28 Vas deferens
29 Spermatic cord
30 Testis – upper pole
31 Pampiniform plexus
32 Corpus spongiosum
33 Urethra
34 Corpus cavernosum
35 Penile fascia
36 Tunica albuginea of penis
37 Deep artery of penis
38 Dorsal vein of penis
39 Investing fascia of thigh – fascia lata

40 Quadratus femoris

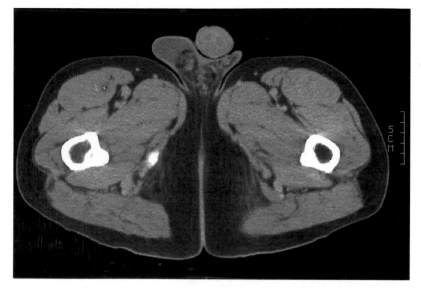

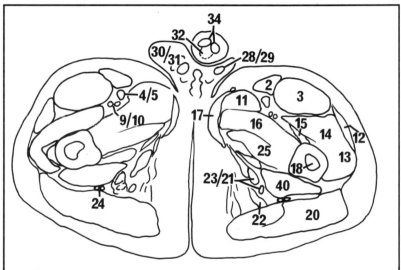

NOTES

This section passes through the anal verge (27) surrounded by the external anal sphincter (26).

It demonstrates well the structure of the penis in transverse section. The penile urethra (33) is surrounded by the corpus spongiosum (32). Above and lateral to this, on either side, are the corpora cavernosa (34). These structures are bound together within the penile fascia (35). The deep artery of the penis (37) is a branch of the internal pudendal artery, which ends in the deep perineal pouch by dividing into the deep and the dorsal arteries of the penis and the artery to the bulb. The deep artery supplies the corpus cavernosum, the dorsal artery supplies the prepuce and glans while the artery to the bulb supplies the corpus spongiosum.

This section also demonstrates the upper pole of the testis (30) surrounded by its tunica albuginea, and also the vas deferens (28) surrounded by the pampiniform plexus (31).

The saphenous nerve (6), a branch of the femoral nerve, is here seen entering the adductor, or subsartorial, canal (Hunter's canal). This is an aponeurotic tunnel in the middle third of the thigh, formed posteriorly by adductor longus (11) and more distally by adductor magnus (25), anterolaterally by vastus medialis (15), and anteromedially by sartorius (2). Its contents are the superficial femoral artery and vein (4, 5), saphenous nerve (6) and nerve to vastus medialis. (See also section 70.)

S3

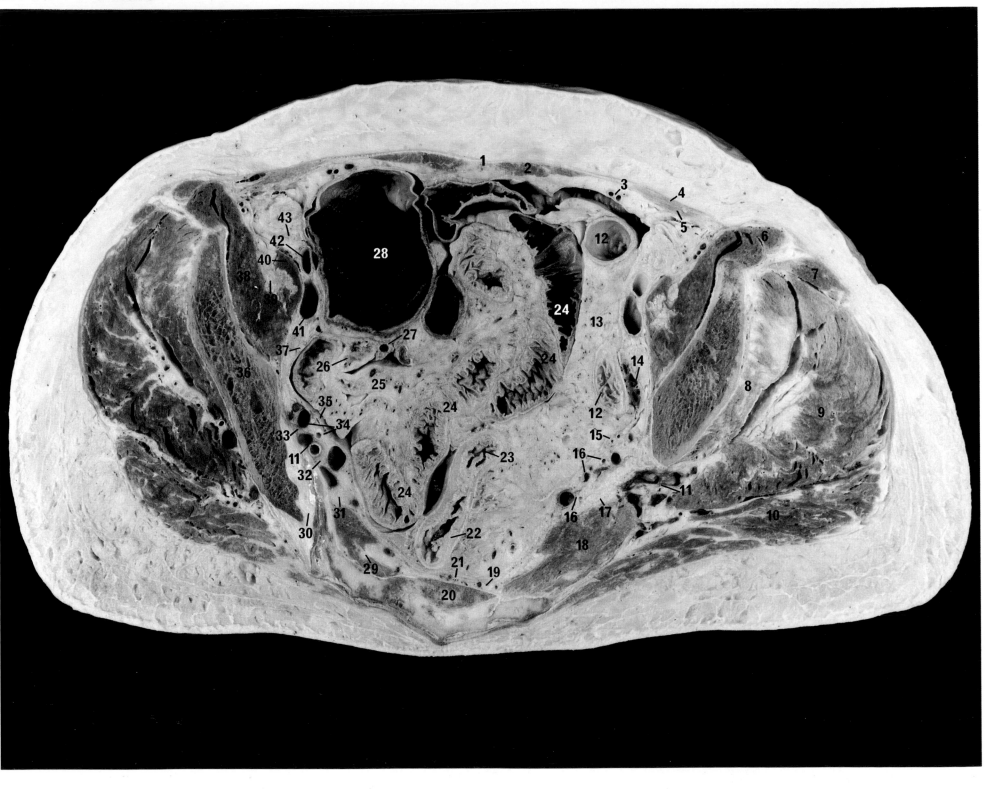

A
R — L
P

1 Linea alba	22 Rectum
2 Rectus abdominis	23 Rectosigmoid junction
3 Inferior epigastric artery and vein	24 Ileum
	25 Mesentery of small bowel
4 Fused aponeurosis of external and internal oblique muscles	26 Right ovary
	27 Right uterine (fallopian) tube
5 Transversus abdominis	28 Caecum
6 Sartorius	29 Ventral ramus of third sacral nerve
7 Tensor fasciae latae	
8 Gluteus minimus	30 Sacro-iliac joint
9 Gluteus medius	31 Ventral ramus of second sacral nerve
10 Gluteus maximus	
11 Superior gluteal artery and vein	32 Ventral ramus of first sacral nerve
	33 Lumbosacral trunk
12 Sigmoid colon	34 Uterine artery and vein
13 Sigmoid mesocolon	35 Right ureter
14 Left ovary	36 Ilium
15 Left ureter	37 Obturator nerve
16 Branches of internal iliac artery and vein	38 Iliacus
	39 Femoral nerve
17 Sciatic nerve	40 Psoas major
18 Piriformis	41 External iliac vein
19 Lateral sacral artery and vein	42 External iliac artery
	43 Lymph node
20 Sacrum third segment	
21 Median sacral artery and vein	44 Uterus (fundus)
	45 Round ligament

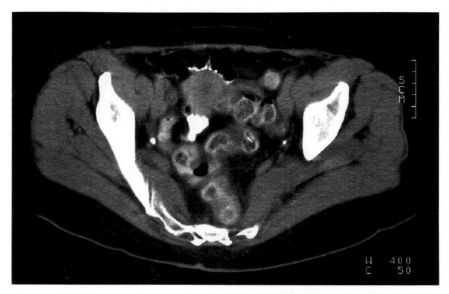

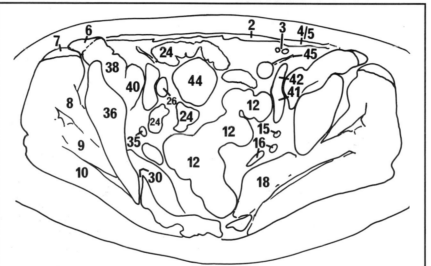

NOTES

This section through the female pelvis transects the third segment of the sacrum (20), which delimits the commencement of the rectum (22) at its junction with the sigmoid colon (23).

The left ovary is seen at (14) and the right ovary at (26); in this elderly subject they are atrophic.

Along the internal iliac vessels (16) lies a rich lymphatic plexus, together with the internal iliac lymph nodes. These receive afferents from all the pelvic viscera, the deeper parts of the perineum and the muscles of the buttock. Their efferents pass through the common iliac nodes.

The sciatic nerve (17) at its origin is lying on piriformis (18). Its important relationships can be traced in subsequent sections as it emerges through the greater sciatic foramen below piriformis to cross, in turn, the obturator internus tendon with its accompanying gemelli, quadratus femoris and, finally, adductor magnus. It is covered superficially by gluteus maximus and is crossed by the long head of the biceps.

Note that a degree of scoliosis in this subject explains the assymetry of the sciatic nerve and other structures on the two sides of this section.

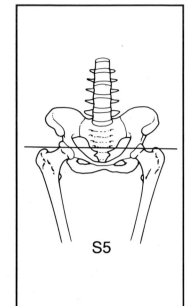

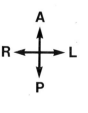

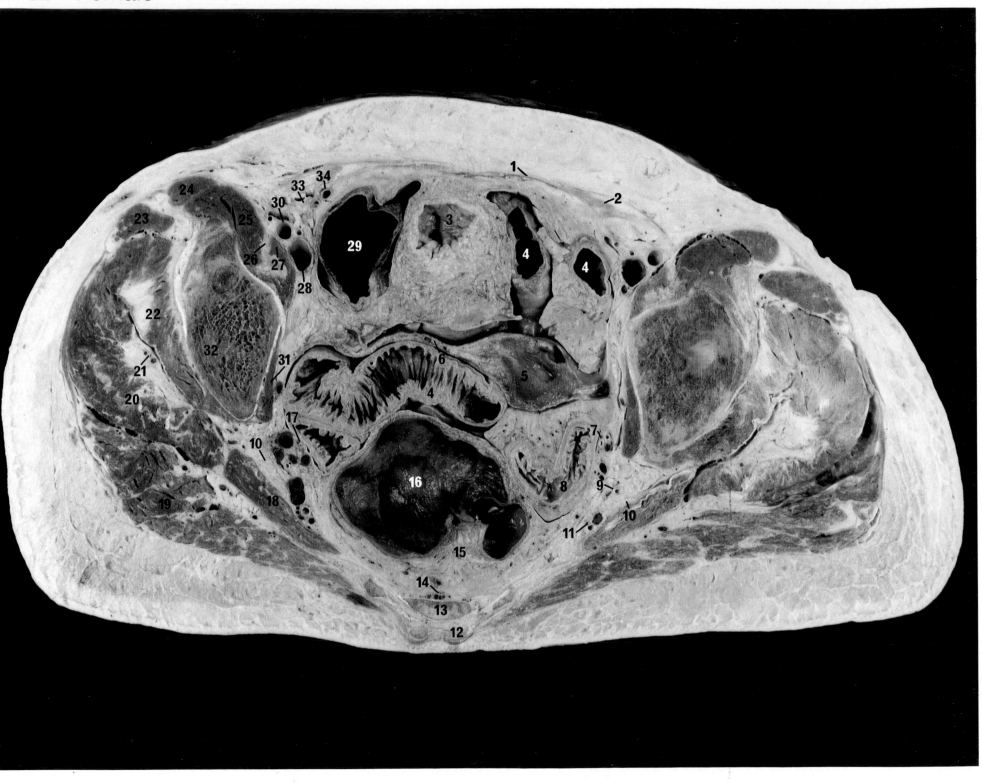

1 Rectus sheath
2 Transversus abdominis
3 Fundus of bladder
4 Ileum
5 Fundus of uterus
6 Broad ligament
7 Left ureter
8 Sigmoid colon
9 Inferior gluteal artery, vein and nerve
10 Sciatic nerve
11 Internal pudendal artery, vein and pudendal nerve
12 Superior sacral cornu
13 Sacrum fifth segment
14 Median sacral artery and vein
15 Mesorectum with superior rectal artery and vein
16 Rectum
17 Right ureter
18 Piriformis
19 Gluteus maximus
20 Gluteus medius
21 Superior gluteal artery and vein
22 Gluteus minimus
23 Tensor fasciae latae
24 Sartorius
25 Iliacus
26 Femoral nerve
27 Psoas major
28 External iliac vein
29 Caecum
30 External iliac artery
31 Obturator internus
32 Ilium
33 Round ligament
34 Inferior epigastric artery and vein

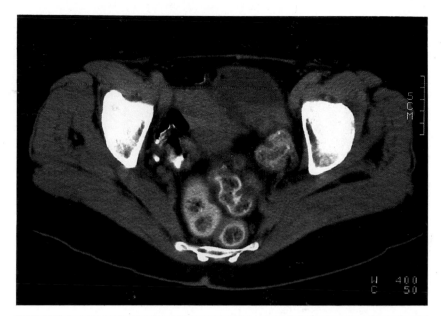

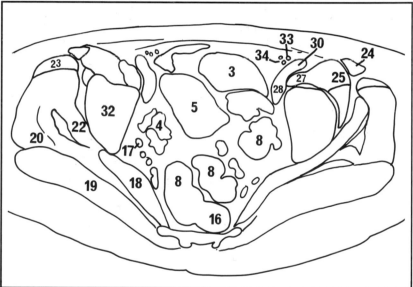

NOTES

This section passes through the lowest, fifth, segment of the sacrum (13) and shaves through the fundus of the bladder (3) and of the uterus (5), together with the upper part of the broad ligament (6).

There is wide normal variation in the relative positions of the pelvic organs. For example, on the CT images the fundus of the uterus was first encountered on the image, section 61. On this CT image, the body of the uterus is traversed. Conversely, the rectosigmoid junction lies at a more caudal level on the CT images than on the sections.

The rectum, from its narrow lumen at its origin, shown in the previous section, has widened into its patulous ampulla (16).

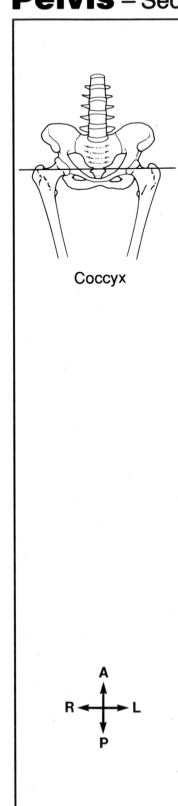

Coccyx

A
R ←→ L
P

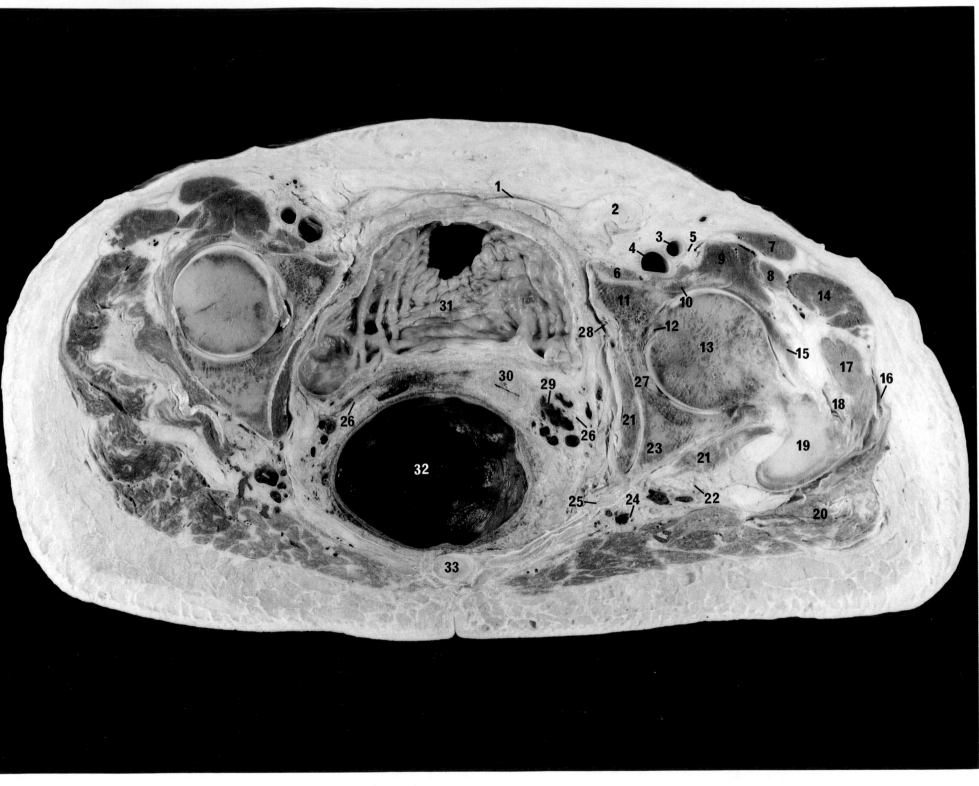

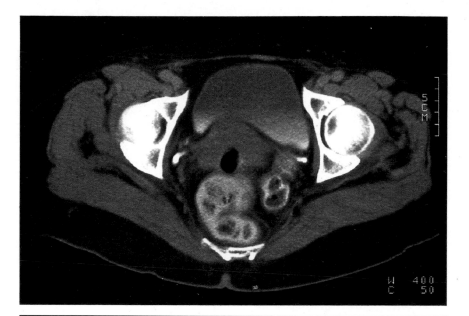

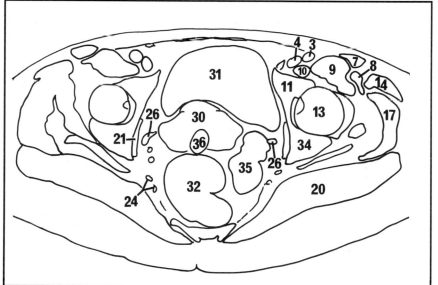

NOTES

This section passes through the coccyx (33) and transects the femoral head (13). In this elderly subject the uterus is atrophic; note the small size of the cervix, here divided through its internal os (30).

Most CT units prepare all female patients undergoing pelvic CT by giving dilute iodinated contrast medium *per rectum*, as here; this renders the lumen of the rectosigmoid opaque. It is also useful if a tampon is inserted into the vagina; the air trapped by its fibres is readily recognized (36). This allows appreciation of the level of the vaginal vault and the external os of the cervix (30), even though neither structure is directly demonstrated.

The uterine artery (29) arises from the internal iliac artery, runs medially on levator ani towards the cervix of the uterus, and crosses above and in front of the ureter (26) above the lateral vaginal fornix to reach the side of the uterus, where it ascends in the broad ligament. The corresponding uterine veins (29), usually two in number, drain a uterine plexus along the lateral side of the uterus within the broad ligament and open into the internal iliac vein. The close relationship between the uterine vessels and the ureter is, of course, of immense importance to the gynaecological surgeon in performing a hysterectomy (see also CT image, section 64).

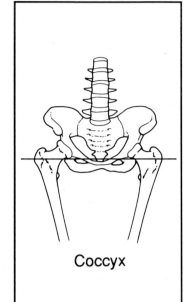

Coccyx

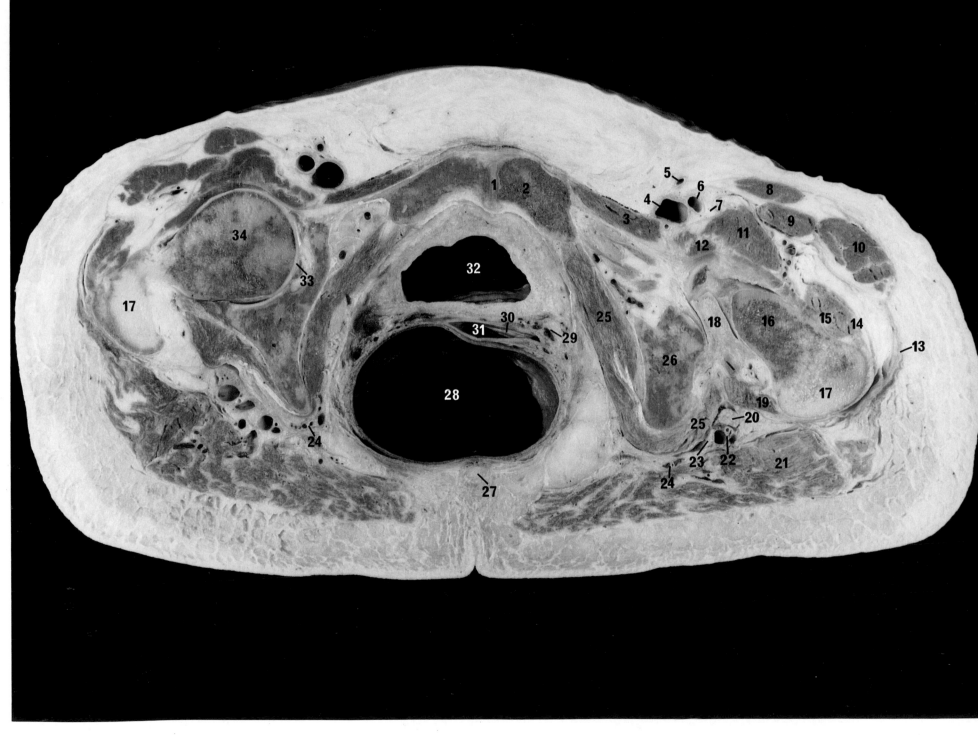

A
R ← → L
P

1 Pubic symphysis
2 Body of pubis
3 Pectineus
4 Femoral vein
5 Great saphenous vein
6 Femoral artery
7 Femoral nerve
8 Sartorius
9 Rectus femoris
10 Tensor fasciae latae
11 Iliacus
12 Psoas major tendon
13 Iliotibial tract
14 Gluteus medius
15 Gluteus minimus
16 Neck of femur
17 Greater trochanter
18 Ischiofemoral ligament
19 Quadratus femoris
20 Sciatic nerve
21 Gluteus maximus
22 Inferior gluteal artery and vein
23 Posterior cutaneous nerve of thigh
24 Internal pudendal artery and vein and pudendal nerve
25 Obturator internus
26 Ischium
27 Coccyx
28 Ampulla of rectum
29 Vaginal artery and vein
30 External os of cervix
31 Vagina
32 Bladder
33 Acetabulum
34 Femoral head

35 Ureter
36 Calcified phleboliths
37 Obturator artery, vein and nerve
38 Ischial spine

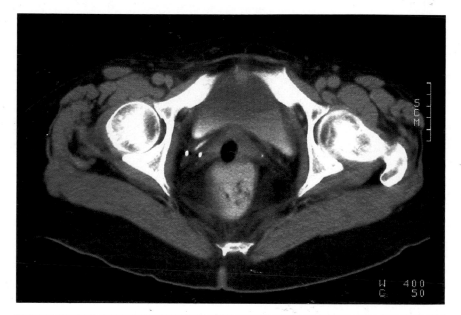

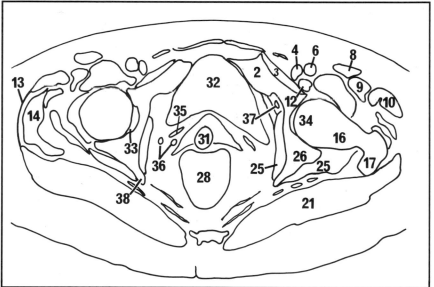

This section traverses the tip of the coccyx (27) and passes through the pubic symphysis in its upper part (1).

Note that the vagina (31) is transected in its upper part so that the external os of the cervix (30) can be seen peeping through with the posterior fornix of the vagina behind it. Alongside the vagina are the vaginal vessels (29). The vaginal artery usually corresponds to the inferior vesical artery in the male and is a branch of the internal iliac artery. It is frequently double or triple. It supplies the vagina as well as the fundus of the bladder and the adjacent part of the rectum, and anastomoses with branches of the uterine artery.

This section shows well the obturator internus muscle (25) as it sweeps around the lesser sciatic foramen with the sciatic nerve (20) lying on its superficial (posterior) face covered posteriorly by the gluteus maximus (21).

Many patients develop small outpouchings, or diverticula, in the extensive plexus of small pelvic veins. These diverticula often contain calcified thrombus to form phleboliths, as demonstrated on the CT image (36). On plain pelvic radiographs these may simulate ureteric calculi.

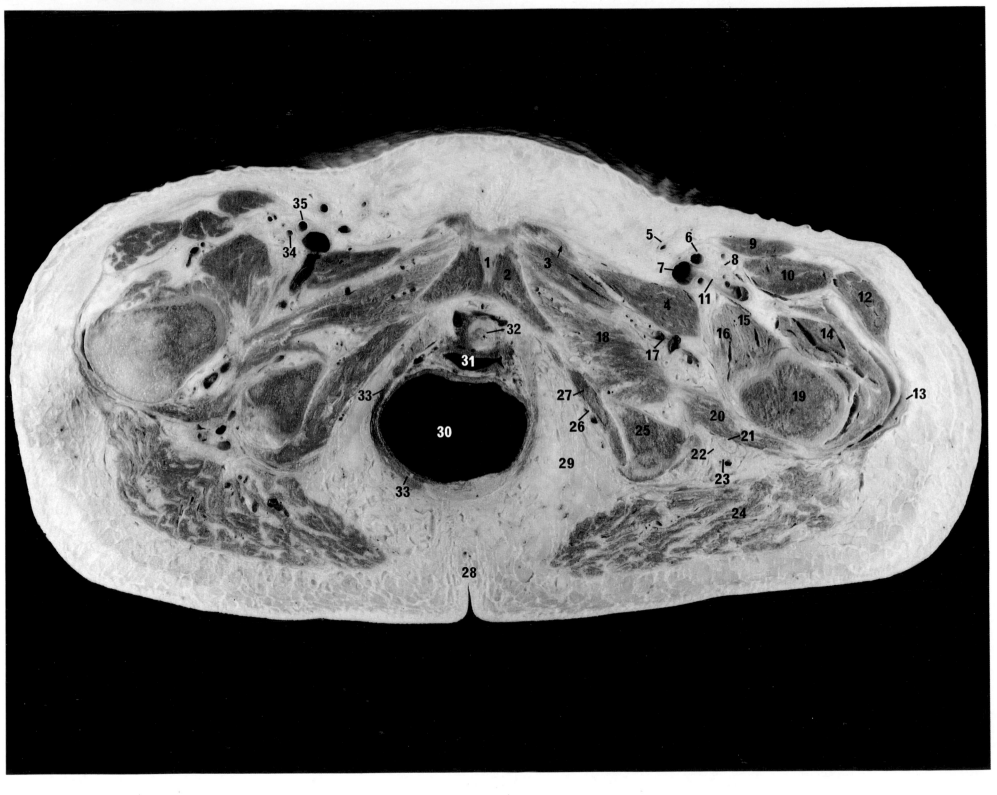

1 Symphysis pubis
2 Body of pubis
3 Adductor brevis, with adductor longus origin (arrowed)
4 Pectineus
5 Great saphenous vein
6 Left femoral artery
7 Femoral vein
8 Femoral nerve
9 Sartorius
10 Rectus femoris
11 Lateral circumflex femoral vein
12 Tensor fasciae latae
13 Iliotibial tract
14 Vastus lateralis
15 Iliacus
16 Psoas major tendon
17 Obturator artery and vein
18 Obturator externus
19 Femur
20 Quadratus femoris
21 Sciatic nerve
22 Posterior cutaneous nerve of thigh
23 Inferior gluteal artery and vein
24 Gluteus maximus
25 Ischial tuberosity
26 Pudendal (Alcock's) canal containing internal pudendal artery and vein and pudendal nerve
27 Obturator internus
28 Natal cleft
29 Ischiorectal fossa
30 Rectum
31 Vagina
32 Urethra
33 Levator ani
34 Right profunda femoris artery
35 Right superficial femoral artery

36 Coccyx
37 Bladder

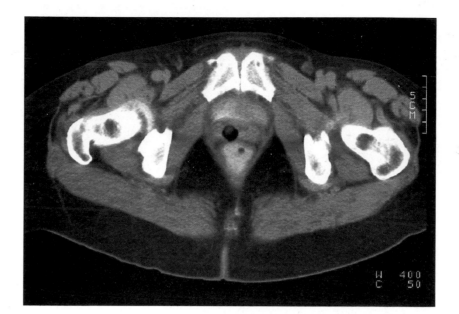

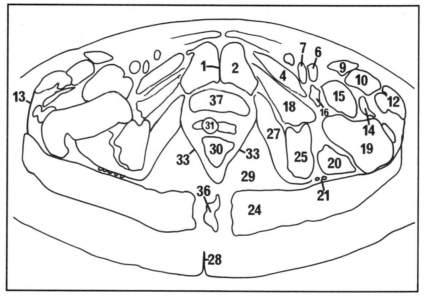

NOTES

This section passes through the upper part of the natal cleft (28) and the body of the pubis (2).

The intimate relationship between the female urethra (32) and vagina (31) is well shown: the former is actually embedded in the anterior wall of the latter.

Unusually, the lateral circumflex femoral vein (11) in this subject arises from the common femoral vein (7); more usually, the circumflex vessels arise from the profunda femoris artery and vein. The right common femoral artery has divided into its profunda (34) and superficial (35) branches. On the left side, the femoral artery (6) has not yet divided.

The anatomy of the ischiorectal fossa (29) is nicely demonstrated. It lies between levator ani (33) and obturator internus (27), on which can be seen the pudendal canal (26) and its contents. (See also section 57.)

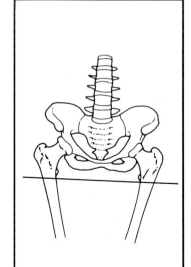

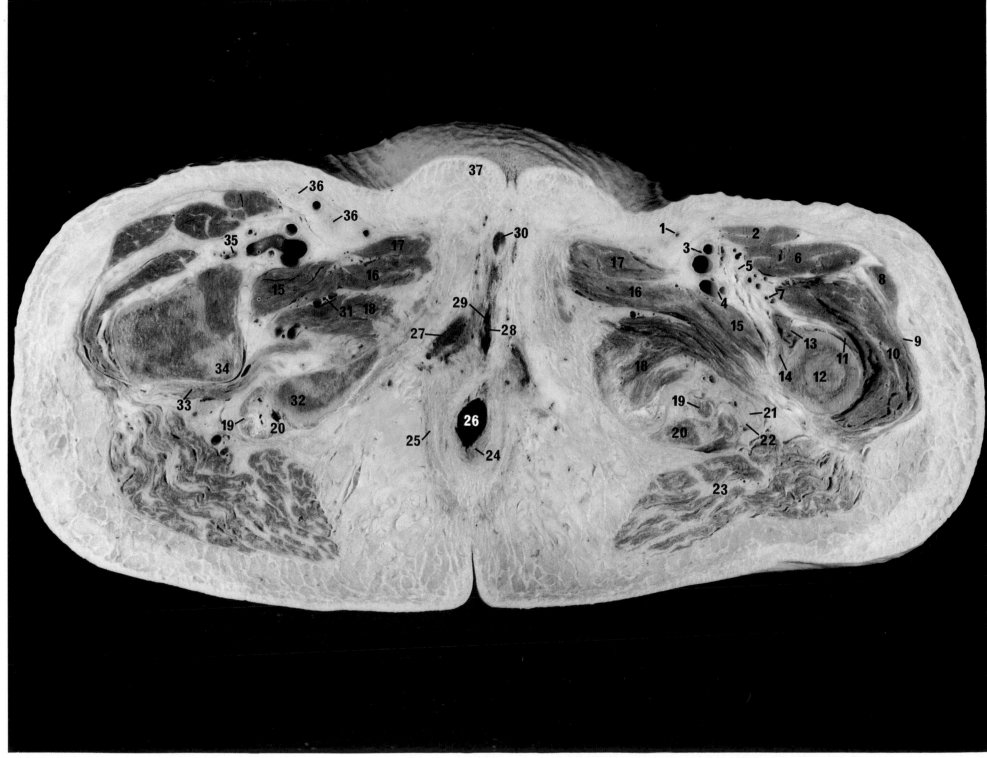

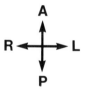

1 Great saphenous vein
2 Sartorius
3 Superficial femoral artery and vein
4 Deep femoral artery and vein
5 Femoral nerve (dividing into branches)
6 Rectus femoris
7 Lateral circumflex femoral artery and vein
8 Tensor fasciae latae
9 Iliotibial tract
10 Vastus lateralis
11 Vastus intermedius
12 Shaft of femur
13 Vastus medialis
14 Psoas major insertion to lesser trochanter with iliacus
15 Pectineus
16 Adductor brevis
17 Adductor longus
18 Adductor magnus
19 Tendon of semimembranosus
20 Origin of semitendinosus and biceps femoris muscles
21 Sciatic nerve
22 Posterior cutaneous nerve of thigh
23 Gluteus maximus
24 External anal sphincter
25 Levator ani
26 Anal canal
27 Crus of clitoris
28 Vaginal orifice
29 Urethral orifice
30 Clitoris
31 Obturator artery, vein and nerve (posterior branch)
32 Ischial tuberosity
33 Quadratus femoris
34 Lesser trochanter of femur
35 Lateral circumflex femoral vein
36 Inguinal lymph node
37 Mons pubis

38 Obturator externus
39 Ischiorectal fossa

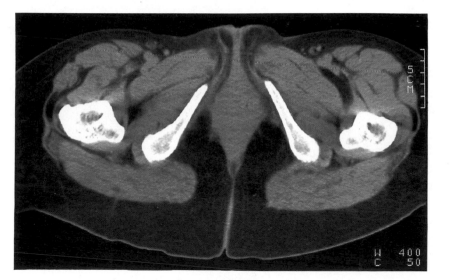

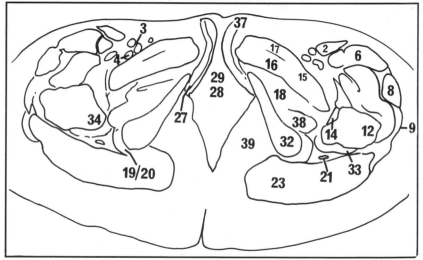

NOTES

This section passes through the mons pubis (37) anteriorly and the anal canal (26) posteriorly. Note the close relationship between the vaginal (28) and urethral (29) orifices.

The sciatic nerve (21), with its accompanying posterior cutaneous nerve of the thigh (22) immediately superficial to it, can now be seen as it lies on quadratus femoris (33).

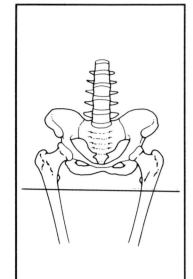

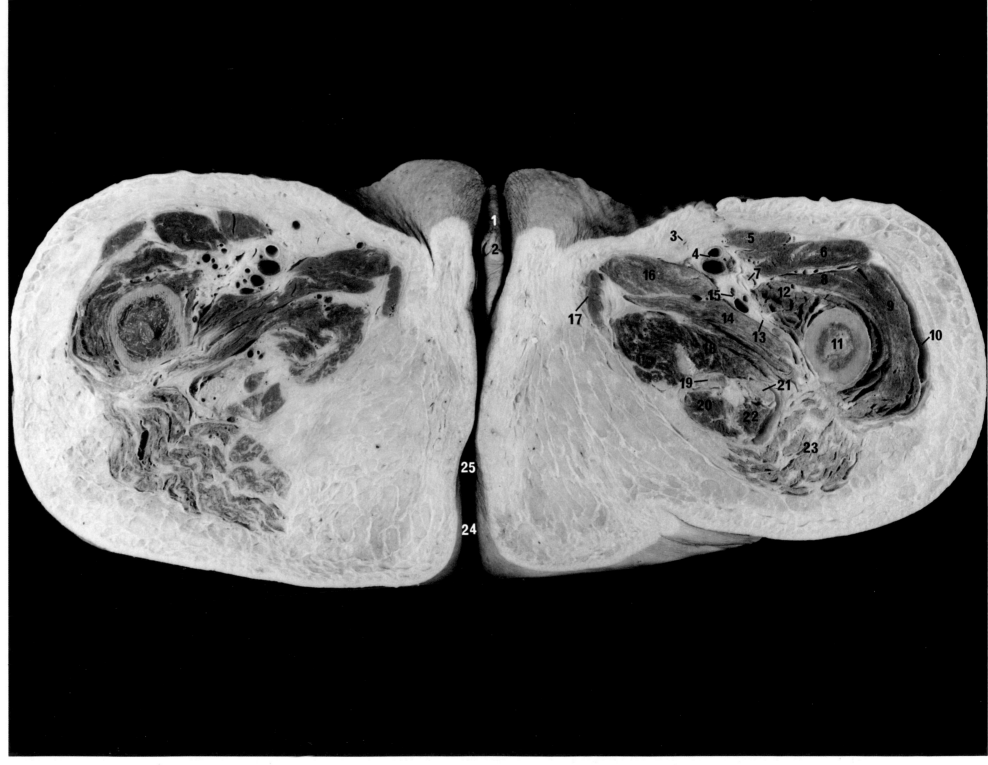

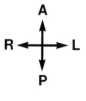

1 Prepuce of clitoris
2 Glans clitoridis
3 Great saphenous vein
4 Superficial femoral artery and vein
5 Sartorius
6 Rectus femoris
7 Femoral nerve (branch to quadratus femoris)
8 Vastus intermedius
9 Vastus lateralis
10 Iliotibial tract
11 Shaft of femur
12 Vastus medialis
13 First perforating artery and vein of profunda femoris artery and vein
14 Adductor brevis
15 Profunda femoris artery and vein
16 Adductor longus
17 Gracilis
18 Adductor magnus
19 Semimembranosus tendon
20 Semitendinosus
21 Sciatic nerve
22 Long head of biceps
23 Gluteus maximus
24 Natal cleft
25 Anal verge

26 Tensor fasciae latae

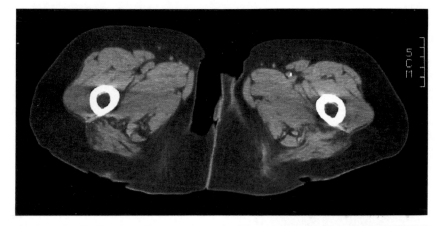

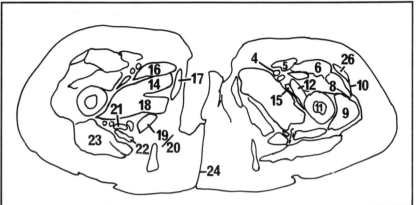

NOTES

This section passes through the upper thigh but demonstrates the prepuce (1) and glans (2) of the clitoris. The anal verge (25) can be seen within the natal cleft (24). The sciatic nerve (21) now lies on adductor magnus (18) and is crossed superficially by the long head of biceps (22).

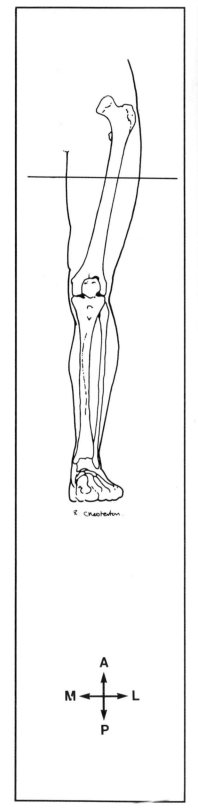

R. Chesterton.

A
M ← → L
P

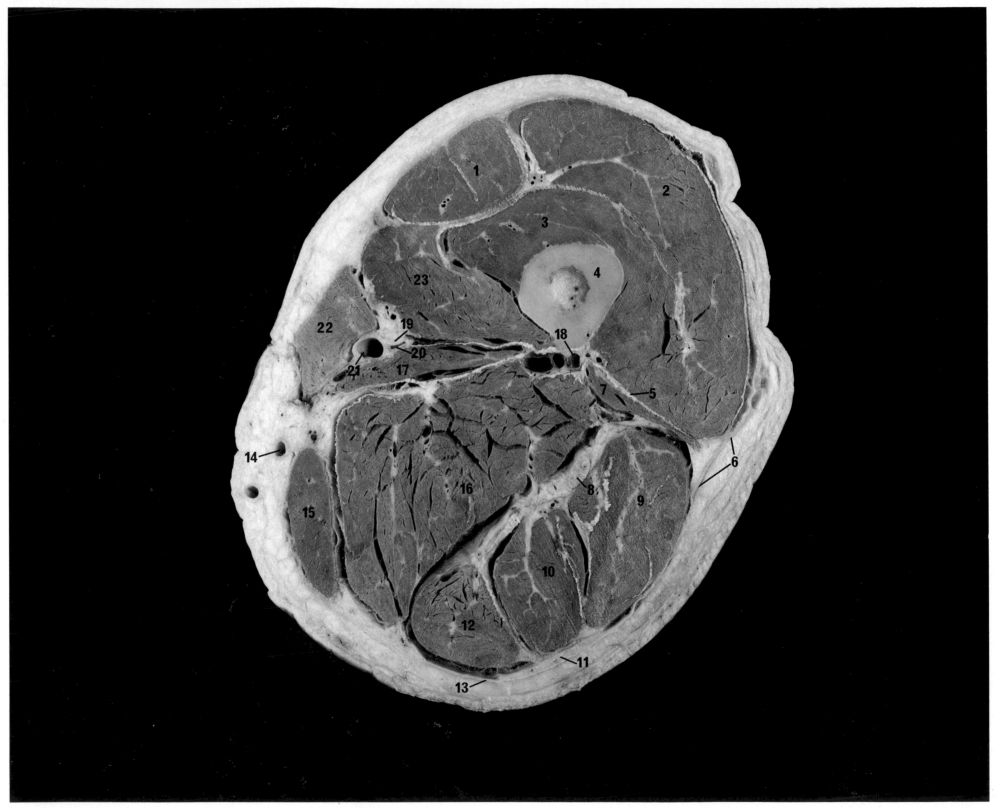

1 Rectus femoris
2 Vastus lateralis
3 Vastus intermedius
4 Femur
5 Lateral intermuscular septum
6 Iliotibial tract
7 Biceps femoris – short head
8 Sciatic nerve
9 Biceps femoris – long head
10 Semitendinosus
11 Posterior cutaneous nerve of thigh
12 Semimembranosus
13 Fascia lata (deep fascia of thigh)
14 Great saphenous vein
15 Gracilis
16 Adductor magnus
17 Adductor longus
18 Profunda femoris artery
19 Saphenous nerve
20 Superficial femoral vein
21 Superficial femoral artery
22 Sartorius
23 Vastus medialis

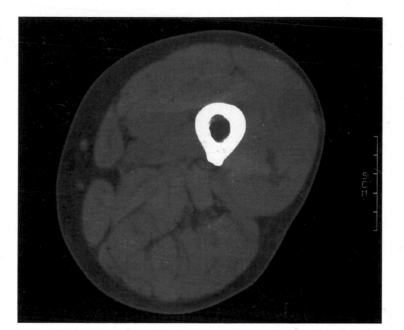

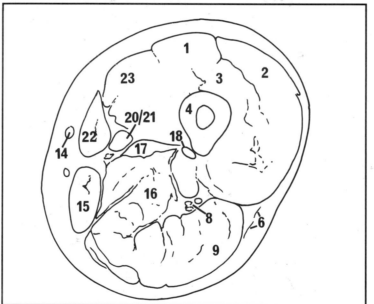

NOTES

This section passes through the upper one third of the thigh and provides a useful view of the three muscular compartments of the thigh:

1. *The anterior compartment* – containing quadriceps femoris, made up of the vasti (2, 3, 23) and rectus femoris (1), supplied by the femoral nerve.
2. *The adductor compartment* – containing the three adductors (of which only adductor magnus (16) and adductor longus (17) are present at this level, brevis having already found insertion into the femoral shaft), together with gracilis (15). These muscles are supplied by the obturator nerve; adductor magnus, in addition, receives innervation from the sciatic nerve.
3. *The posterior compartment* – contains the hamstrings – the biceps with its long and short heads (9 and 7 respectively), semitendinosus (10) and semimembranosus (12), all supplied by the sciatic nerve (8).

Sartorius (22) lies in a separate fascial sheath.

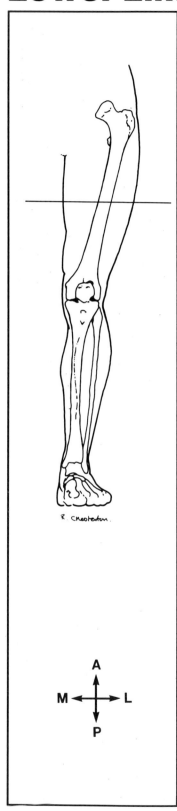

R. Chesterton

A
M ← → L
P

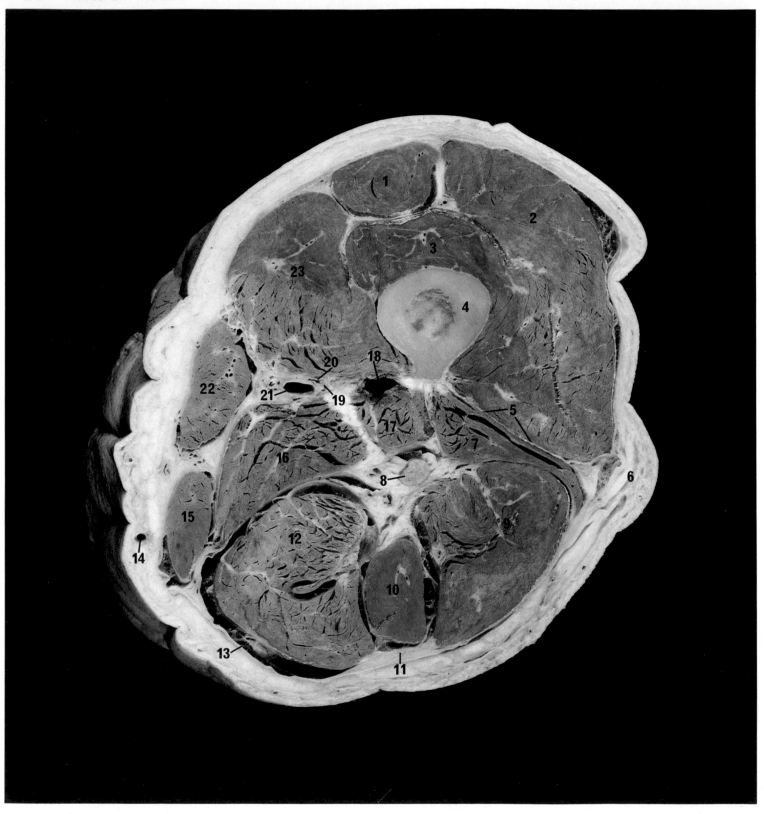

1 Rectus femoris
2 Vastus lateralis
3 Vastus intermedius
4 Femur
5 Lateral intermuscular septum
6 Iliotibial tract
7 Biceps femoris – short head
8 Sciatic nerve
9 Biceps femoris – long head
10 Semitendinosus
11 Posterior cutaneous nerve of thigh
12 Semimembranosus
13 Fascia lata (deep fascia of thigh)
14 Great saphenous vein
15 Gracilis
16 Adductor magnus medial part
17 Adductor magnus lateral part
18 Profunda femoris artery
19 Saphenous nerve
20 Superficial femoral vein
21 Superficial femoral artery
22 Sartorius
23 Vastus medialis

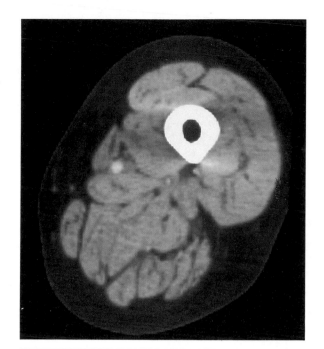

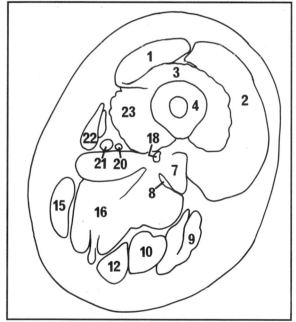

NOTES

This section passes through the mid-shaft of the femur (4).

A bolus intravenous injection of iodinated contrast material has been given before this CT image was taken; hence the femoral artery (21) and profunda femoris artery (18) are clearly seen.

Note that, at this level, adductor magnus is dividing into two sections. Its lateral part (17), which arises from the ischial ramus, forms a broad aponeurosis which inserts along the linea aspera along the posterior border of the femoral shaft (4). The medial part (16), which arises mainly from the ischial tuberosity, descends almost vertically to a tendinous attachment to the adductor tubercle of the medial condyle of the femur. Between the two parts distally is the osseo-aponeurotic adductor hiatus, which admits the femoral vessels to the popliteal fossa.

Being a composite muscle, adductor magnus also has a composite nerve supply; the medial part is innervated by the tibial division of the sciatic nerve (8), the lateral part by the obturator nerve.

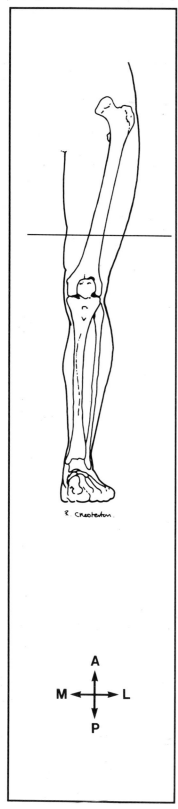

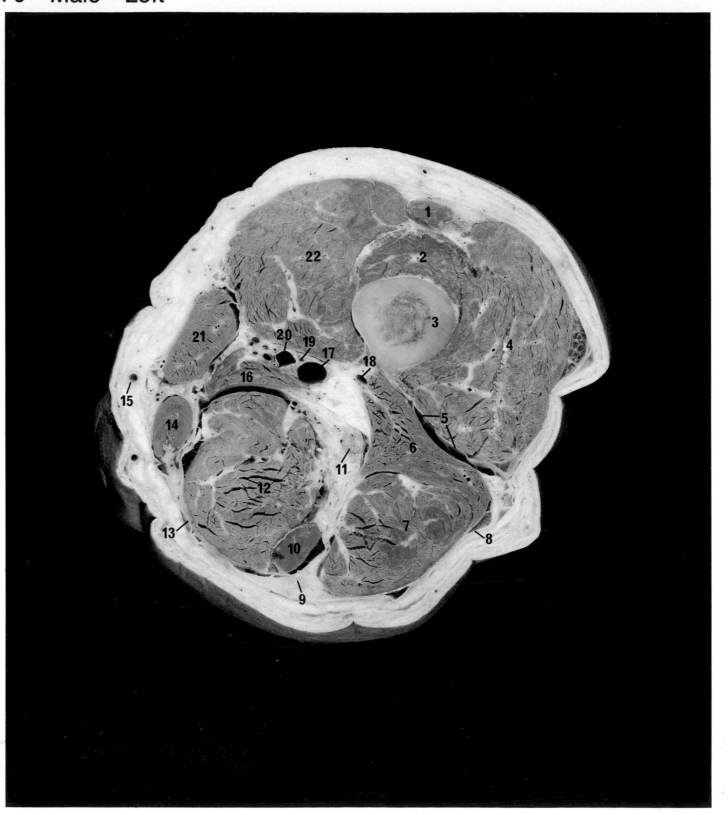

1 Rectus femoris
2 Vastus intermedius
3 Femur
4 Vastus lateralis
5 Lateral intermuscular septum
6 Biceps femoris – short head
7 Biceps femoris – long head
8 Iliotibial tract
9 Posterior cutaneous nerve of thigh
10 Semitendinosus
11 Sciatic nerve
12 Semimembranosus
13 Fascia lata (deep fascia of thigh)
14 Gracilis
15 Great saphenous vein
16 Adductor magnus
17 Superficial femoral vein
18 Profunda femoris artery and vein
19 Saphenous nerve
20 Superficial femoral artery
21 Sartorius
22 Vastus medialis

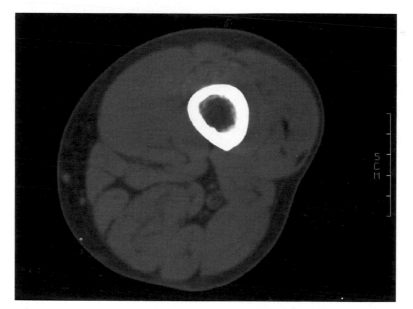

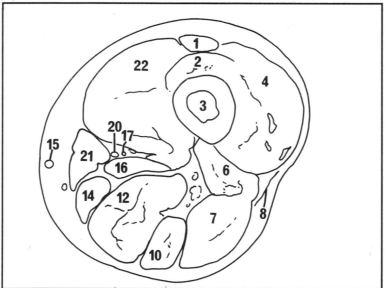

NOTES

This section transects the lower third of the thigh.

This and the previous two sections demonstrate the anatomy of the adductor or subsartorial canal (Hunter's canal). This is formed as a triangular aponeurotic tunnel, which leads from the femoral triangle above to the popliteal fossa below, via the hiatus in adductor magnus. The canal lies between sartorius (21) anteromedially, adductor longus and, more distally, adductor magnus (16) posteriorly, and vastus medialis (22) anterolaterally. Its contents are the superficial femoral artery (20) and vein (17), the saphenous nerve (19) and also the nerve to vastus medialis, until this enters and supplies this muscle.

John Hunter (1728–1793) described ligation of the femoral artery within this canal in the treatment of popliteal aneurysm, and his name has been eponymously attached to the canal.

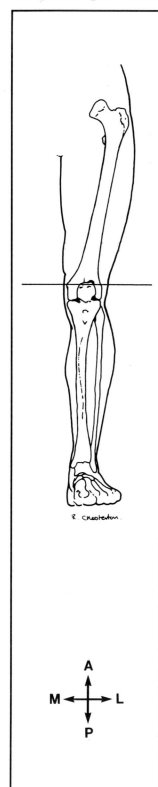

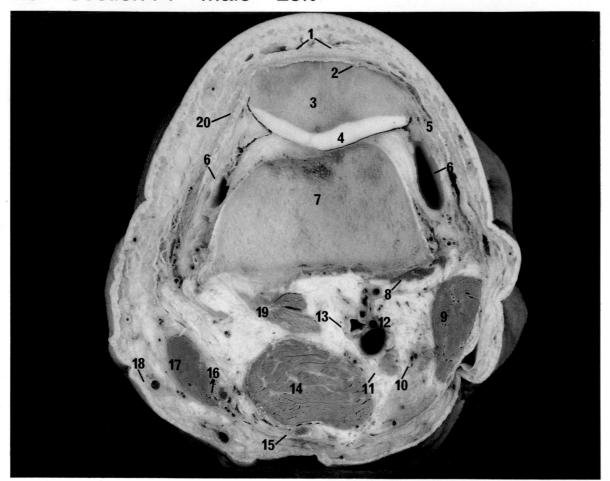

1 Prepatellar bursa
2 Tendon of quadriceps femoris
3 Patella
4 Articular cartilage of patella
5 Tendon of vastus lateralis
6 Capsule of knee joint
7 Femur
8 Plantaris origin
9 Biceps femoris
10 Common peroneal nerve
11 Tibial nerve
12 Popliteal vein
13 Popliteal artery
14 Semimembranosus
15 Semitendinosus
16 Gracilis tendon
17 Sartorius
18 Great saphenous vein
19 Gastrocnemius
20 Tendon of vastus medialis

21 Vastus medialis
22 Vastus lateralis

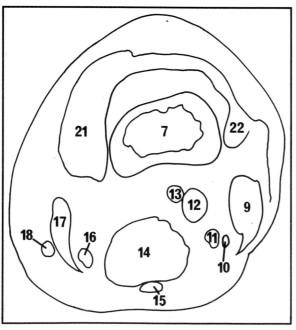

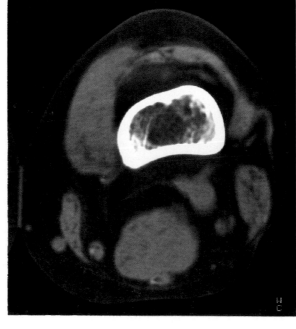

NOTES

This section passes through the upper part of the patella (3) and the femur just as this widens into its condyles (7). The CT image is at a more proximal level, immediately above the patella.

Note how the lateral portion of the patella (3) has a larger and flatter articular surface than the medial. This, together with the low insertion of vastus medialis (20) into the medial side of the patella, helps to prevent lateral dislocation of the patella.

The sciatic nerve has now divided into the common peroneal nerve (10) and the tibial nerve (11): the latter is usually about twice the size of the former. Division usually takes place just proximal to the knee, but the sciatic nerve may divide anywhere along its course. Indeed, its division may take place at the sciatic plexus, when the common peroneal nerve usually pierces the piriformis muscle in the greater sciatic foramen and the tibial division emerges caudal to this muscle.

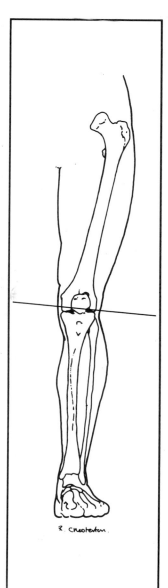

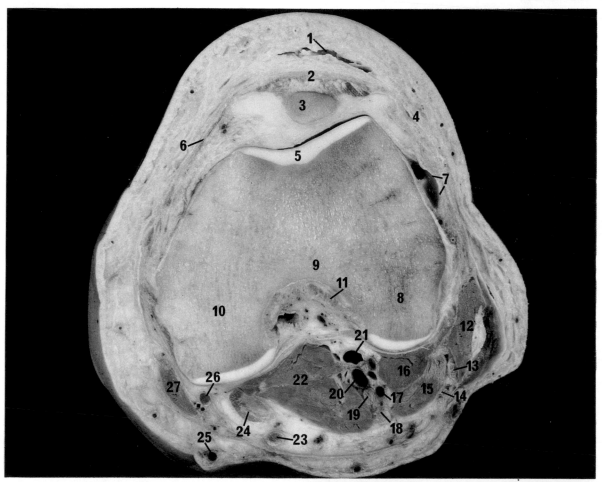

1 **Prepatellar bursa**
2 **Ligamentum patellae**
3 **Patella**
4 **Lateral patellar retinaculum**
5 **Articular cartilage of femur**
6 **Medial patellar retinaculum**
7 **Capsule of knee joint**
8 **Lateral condyle of femur**
9 **Intercondylar fossa**
10 **Medial condyle of femur**
11 **Anterior cruciate ligament**
12 **Biceps femoris**
13 **Common peroneal nerve**
14 **Sural communicating nerve**
15 **Gastrocnemius – lateral head**
16 **Plantaris**
17 **Small saphenous vein – termination**
18 **Sural nerve**
19 **Tibial nerve**
20 **Popliteal vein**
21 **Popliteal artery**
22 **Gastrocnemius – medial head**
23 **Semitendinosus tendon**
24 **Semimembranosus tendon**
25 **Great saphenous vein**
26 **Gracilis tendon**
27 **Sartorius**

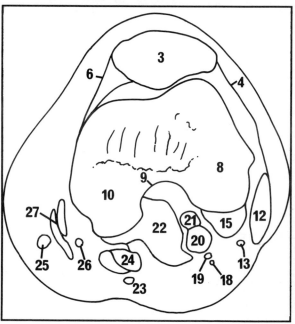

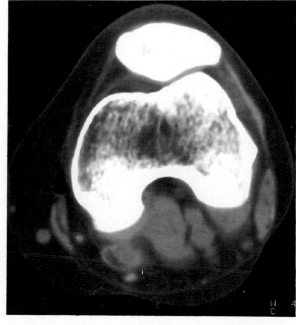

NOTES

This section passes through the distal extremity of the patella (3) and the femoral condyles (8, 10).

The anterior cruciate ligament (11) arises from the intercondylar fossa (9) of the femur laterally and more proximally than the posterior cruciate ligament, whose attachment will be seen in the next section. The anterior cruciate ligament passes downwards and forwards laterally to the posterior cruciate ligament, to attach to the anterior intercondylar area of the tibia.

The small saphenous vein (17), which will be seen in later sections as it lies in the superficial fascia of the back of the calf, has here pierced the deep fascia of the popliteal fossa and is about to drain into the popliteal vein (20).

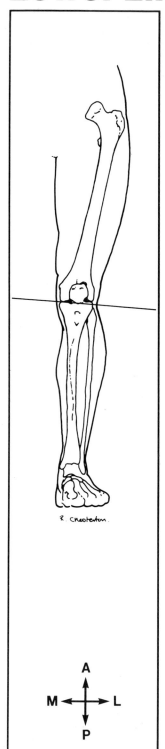

R. Chesterton

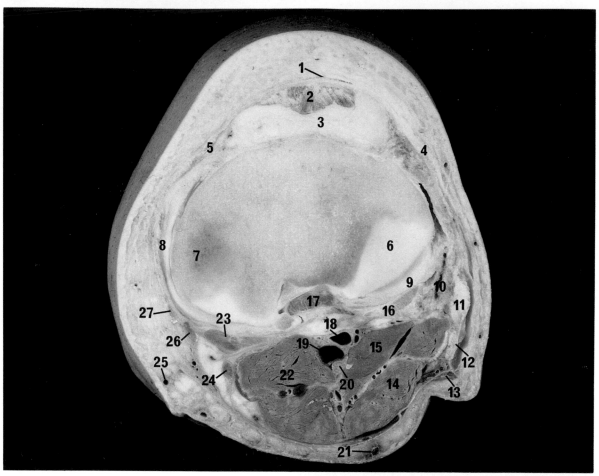

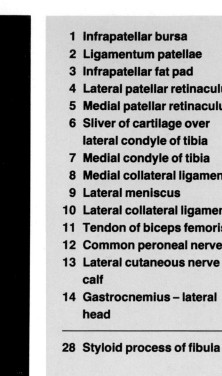

1	Infrapatellar bursa	15	Plantaris
2	Ligamentum patellae	16	Popliteus
3	Infrapatellar fat pad	17	Posterior cruciate ligament
4	Lateral patellar retinaculum	18	Popliteal artery
5	Medial patellar retinaculum	19	Popliteal vein
6	Sliver of cartilage over lateral condyle of tibia	20	Tibial nerve
		21	Small saphenous vein
7	Medial condyle of tibia	22	Gastrocnemius – medial head
8	Medial collateral ligament		
9	Lateral meniscus	23	Semimembranosus tendon
10	Lateral collateral ligament	24	Semitendinosus tendon
11	Tendon of biceps femoris	25	Great saphenous vein
12	Common peroneal nerve	26	Gracilis tendon
13	Lateral cutaneous nerve of calf	27	Sartorius tendon
14	Gastrocnemius – lateral head		

28 Styloid process of fibula

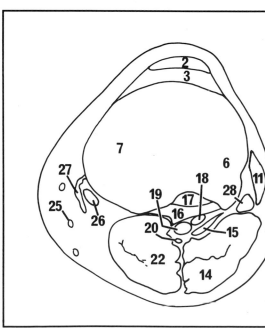

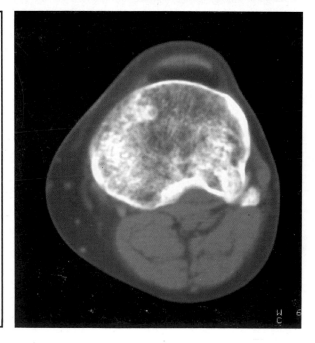

NOTES

This section passes through the tibial condyles (6, 7).

The posterior cruciate ligament (17) is here finding attachment to the posterior intercondylar area of the proximal articular surface of the tibia.

The popliteus tendon (16), which arises from the femur in a depression immediately distal to the lateral epicondyle, passes between the lateral meniscus (9) and the lateral collateral ligament of the knee (10). In contrast, the medial collateral ligament (8) is closely applied to the medial meniscus, which lies just proximal to this plane of section. This tethering of the medial meniscus probably accounts for the much higher incidence of tears of the medial compared with the lateral meniscus.

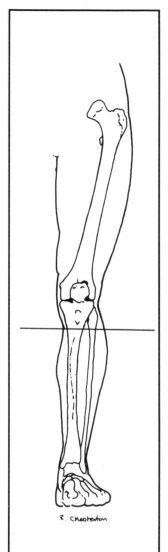

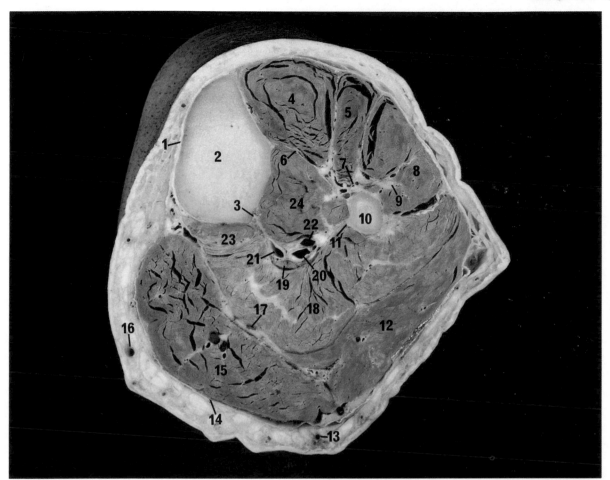

1 Subcutaneous surface of tibia
2 Tibia
3 Vertical ridge of tibia
4 Tibialis anterior
5 Extensor digitorum longus
6 Interosseous membrane
7 Anterior tibial artery and vein with deep peroneal nerve
8 Peroneus longus
9 Superficial peroneal nerve
10 Fibula
11 Medial crest of fibula
12 Gastrocnemius – lateral head
13 Small saphenous vein
14 Deep fascia of calf
15 Gastrocnemius – medial head
16 Great saphenous vein
17 Plantaris tendon
18 Soleus
19 Tibial nerve
20 Posterior tibial artery
21 Posterior tibial vein
22 Peroneal artery
23 Popliteus
24 Tibialis posterior

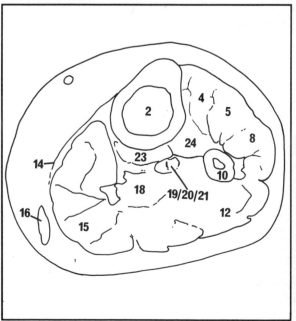

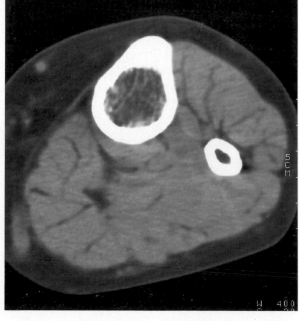

NOTES

This section traverses the proximal end of the tibial shaft (2) and the shaft of the fibula (10) immediately distal to the neck of the fibula.

At this level the common peroneal nerve, which sweeps round the neck of the fibula deep to peroneus longus (8), has divided into its superficial peroneal (9) and deep peroneal (7) branches. The superficial peroneal nerve lies deep to peroneus longus. The deep peroneal nerve passes obliquely forwards deep to extensor digitorum longus (5) to descend with the anterior tibial vessels (7).

The tendon of plantaris (17) lies in a well defined tissue plane between soleus (18) and gastrocnemius (12, 15). Fluid enters this plane following rupture of a semimembranosus bursa (Baker's cyst).

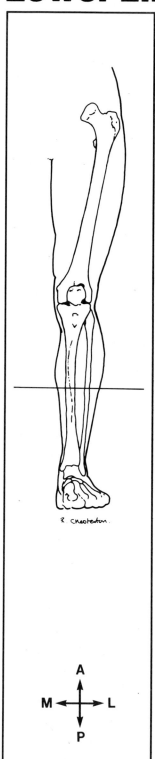

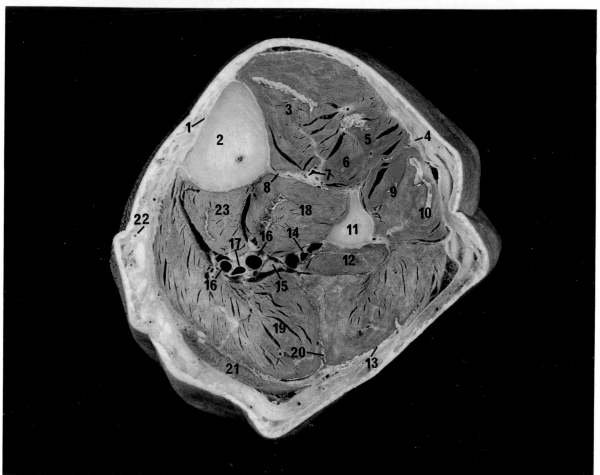

1 Subcutaneous border of tibia
2 Tibia
3 Tibialis anterior
4 Superficial peroneal nerve
5 Extensor digitorum longus
6 Extensor hallucis longus
7 Anterior tibial artery and vein with deep peroneal nerve
8 Interosseous membrane
9 Peroneus brevis
10 Peroneus longus
11 Fibula
12 Flexor hallucis longus
13 Deep fascia of calf
14 Peroneal artery with venae comitantes
15 Tibial nerve
16 Venae comitantes of posterior tibial artery
17 Posterior tibial artery
18 Tibialis posterior
19 Soleus
20 Plantaris tendon
21 Gastrocnemius
22 Great saphenous vein
23 Flexor digitorum longus

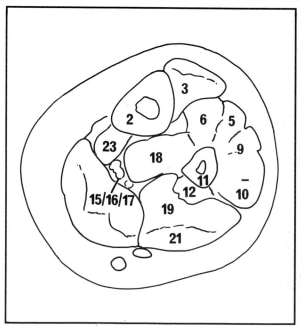

A
M ←→ L
P

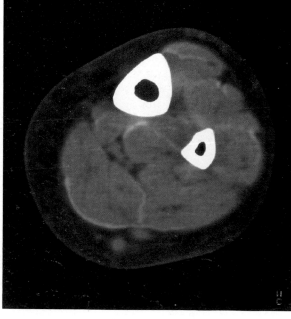

NOTES

This section traverses the mid calf.

Note that the whole of the anteromedial aspect of the shaft of the tibia (1) is subcutaneous, covered only by skin, superficial fascia and periosteum, and crossed, in its lower part, only by the great saphenous vein (22) and saphenous nerve.

The neurovascular bundle of the anterior tibial vessels and deep peroneal nerve (7), having descended first between extensor digitorum longus (5) and tibialis anterior (3), now runs between the latter and extensor hallucis longus (6) as this takes origin from the anterior aspect of the fibular shaft (11).

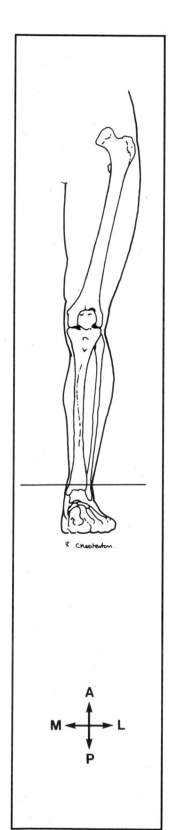

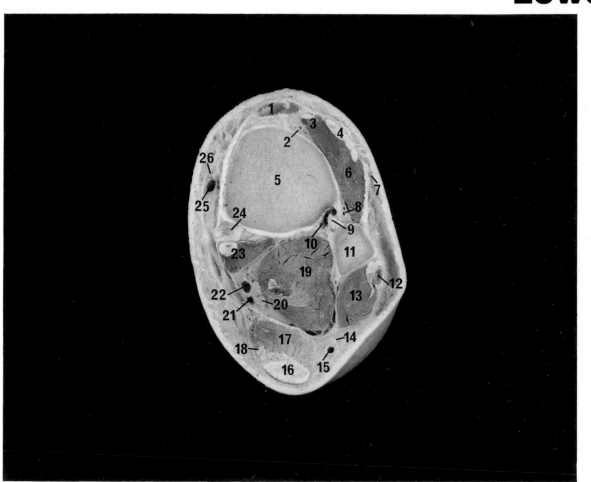

1. Tibialis anterior tendon
2. Anterior tibial artery with venae comitantes and deep peroneal nerve
3. Extensor hallucis longus and tendon
4. Extensor digitorum longus tendon
5. Tibia
6. Peroneus tertius
7. Superficial peroneal nerve
8. Perforating branch of peroneal artery
9. Inferior tibiofibular joint (interosseous ligament)
10. Peroneal artery
11. Fibula
12. Peroneus longus tendon
13. Peroneus brevis
14. Sural nerve
15. Small saphenous vein
16. Tendo calcaneus (Achilles tendon)
17. Soleus
18. Plantaris tendon
19. Flexor hallucis longus
20. Tibial nerve
21. Posterior tibial vein
22. Posterior tibial artery
23. Flexor digitorum longus and tendon
24. Tibialis posterior tendon
25. Great saphenous vein
26. Saphenous nerve

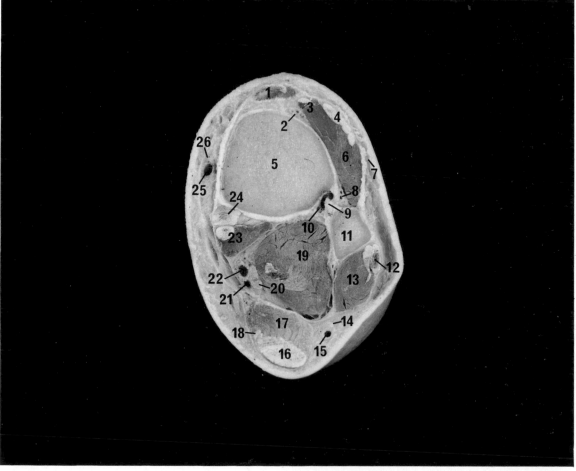

A
M ←→ L
P

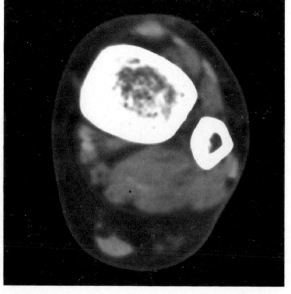

NOTES

This section passes immediately above the ankle joint at the level of the inferior tibiofibular joint (9). This is the only fibrous joint, apart from the skull sutures, and represents, in fact, the thickened distal extremity of the interosseous membrane. (See also section 77.)

At this level, gastroncnemius has already become tendinous (16), although soleus (17) still displays muscle fibres. A little more distally this too will become tendinous and fuse into the tendo calcaneus (tendo Achilles).

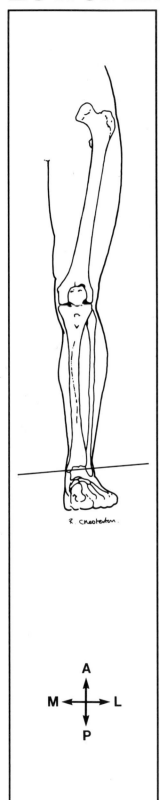

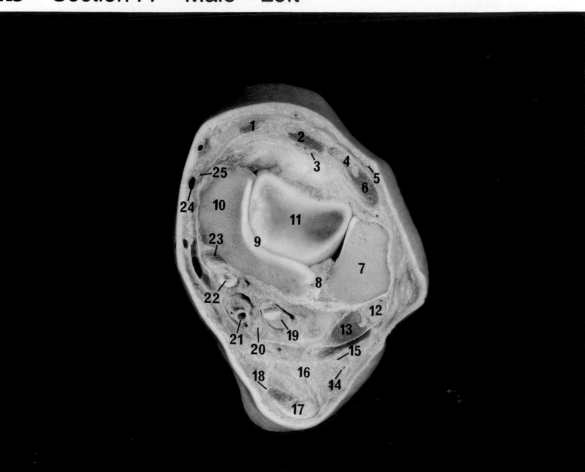

1 **Tibialis anterior tendon**
2 **Extensor hallucis longus and tendon**
3 **Anterior tibial artery and venae comitantes with deep peroneal nerve**
4 **Extensor digitorum tendon**
5 **Superficial peroneal nerve**
6 **Peroneus tertius and tendon**
7 **Lateral malleolus**
8 **Inferior tibiofibular joint**
9 **Ankle joint**
10 **Medial malleolus**
11 **Talus**
12 **Peroneus brevis tendon**
13 **Peroneus longus**
14 **Small saphenous vein**
15 **Sural nerve**
16 **Fat**
17 **Tendo calcaneus**
18 **Plantaris tendon**
19 **Flexor hallucis longus tendon**
20 **Tibial nerve**
21 **Posterior tibial artery with venae comitantes**
22 **Flexor digitorum longus tendon**
23 **Tibialis posterior tendon**
24 **Great saphenous vein**
25 **Saphenous nerve**

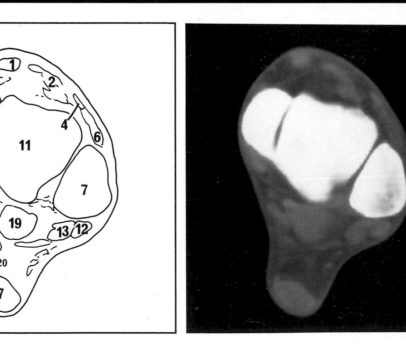

NOTES

This section passes through the ankle joint (9) and the inferior tibiofibular joint (8). Note that this section illustrates the fibrous nature of the inferior tibiofibular joint.

Peroneus brevis (12) and peroneus longus (13) pass behind the lateral malleolus (7) of the fibula and will groove the bone a little more distally to form the malleolar fossa.

This section demonstrates the order of structures which pass behind the medial malleolus (10). These are, from the medial to the lateral side, the tendon of tibialis posterior (23), the tendon of flexor digitorum longus (22), the posterior tibial artery with its venae comitantes (21), the tibial nerve (20) and, most laterally, the tendon of flexor hallucis longus (19).

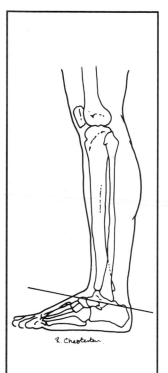

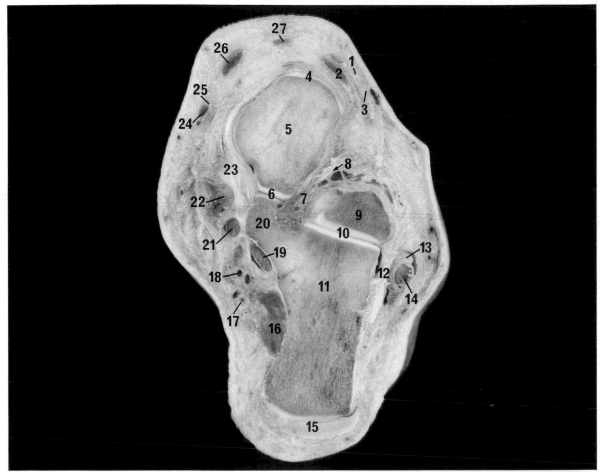

1. Extensor digitorum longus tendon
2. Extensor digitorum brevis
3. Peroneus tertius tendon
4. Talocalcaneonavicular joint (anterior talonavicular part)
5. Head of talus
6. Talocalcaneonavicular joint (posterior part)
7. Interosseous talocalcanean ligament
8. Sulcus tali (arrowed)
9. Lateral process of talus
10. Talocalcanean (subtalar) joint
11. Calcaneus
12. Capsule of talocalcanean joint
13. Peroneus brevis tendon
14. Peroneus longus tendon
15. Tendo Achilles
16. Flexor accessorius
17. Lateral plantar neurovascular bundle
18. Medial plantar neurovascular bundle
19. Flexor hallucis longus tendon
20. Sustentaculum tali
21. Flexor digitorum longus tendon
22. Tibialis posterior tendon
23. Deltoid ligament of ankle
24. Great saphenous vein
25. Saphenous nerve
26. Tibialis anterior tendon
27. Extensor hallucis longus tendon

28. Tibia
29. Medial malleolus
30. Abductor hallucis
31. Abductor digiti minimi

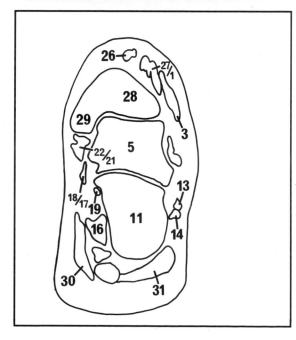

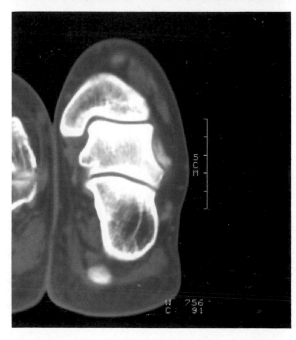

NOTES

This section passes through the head (5) and lateral process (9) of the talus and the calcaneus (11). The CT image is in a more coronal plane, hence the tibia (28) is seen with its articulation with the talus (5).

The tendon of flexor hallucis longus (19) passes behind the sustentaculum tali (20) and, more distally, grooves its inferior aspect. The sulcus tali (8), with its corresponding sulcus calcanei, forms the sinus tarsi and contains the strong interosseous talocalcanean ligament.

The talocalcanean joint (10), also termed the subtalar joint, lies between the convex posterior facet on the upper surface of the calcaneus and the concave posterior facet on the inferior surface of the talus. The talocalcaneonavicular joint is complex. It is formed by the rounded head of the talus (5) which fits into the concavity on the posterior aspect of the navicular, the upper surface of the plantar calcaneonavicular ligament (the spring ligament), which runs between the sustentaculum tali and the inferior aspect of the navicular, and the anterior and middle facets for the talus on the calcaneus. The anterior and posterior portions of this joint are shown at (4) and (6).

A considerable degree of inversion and eversion of the foot takes place at the talocalcanean and talocalcaneonavicular joints.

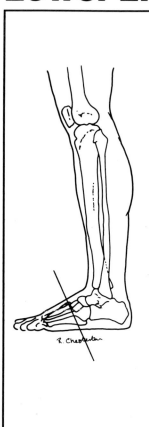

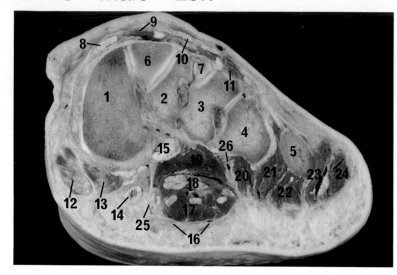

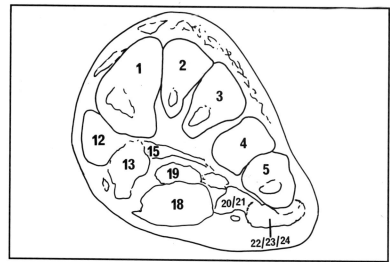

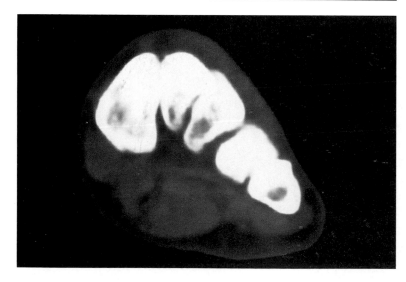

1 First metatarsal
2 Second metatarsal
3 Third metatarsal
4 Fourth metatarsal
5 Fifth metatarsal
6 Medial cuneiform
7 Fragment of lateral cuneiform
8 Extensor hallucis longus tendon
9 Extensor hallucis brevis
10 Extensor digitorum longus tendon
11 Extensor digitorum brevis
12 Abductor hallucis
13 Flexor hallucis brevis
14 Flexor hallucis longus tendon
15 Peroneus longus tendon
16 Plantar aponeurosis
17 Flexor digitorum brevis
18 Flexor digitorum longus tendon
19 Adductor hallucis (oblique head)
20 Second plantar interosseous
21 Third plantar interosseous
22 Flexor digiti minimi
23 Opponens digiti minimi
24 Abductor digiti minimi
25 Medial plantar artery and nerve
26 Lateral plantar artery and nerve

NOTES

This section of the lower limb passes through the forefoot and the bases of the metatarsal bones. It demonstrates the appearance of the transverse arch of the foot.

The tendon of peroneus longus (15), having grooved the inferior aspect of the cuboid, passes forward and medially to insert into the inferolateral aspect of the medial cuneiform (6) and the base of the first metatarsal (1). The sling-like action of this tendon helps maintain the transverse arch.

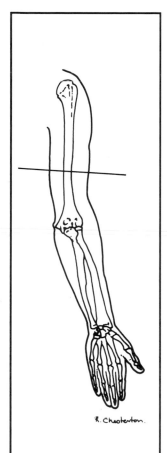

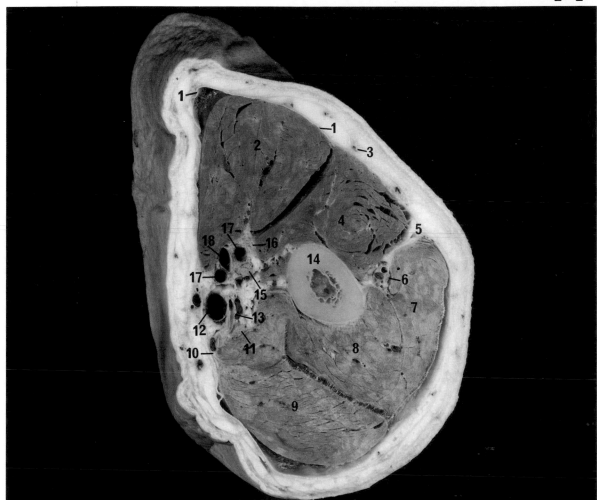

1 Deep fascia of arm
2 Biceps
3 Cephalic vein
4 Brachialis
5 Lateral intermuscular septum
6 Radial nerve with profunda brachii artery and vein
7 Triceps – lateral head
8 Triceps – medial head
9 Triceps – long head
10 Medial intermuscular septum
11 Ulnar nerve
12 Basilic vein
13 Superior ulnar collateral artery and vein
14 Humerus shaft
15 Median nerve
16 Musculocutaneous nerve
17 Venae comitantes of brachial artery
18 Brachial artery

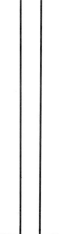

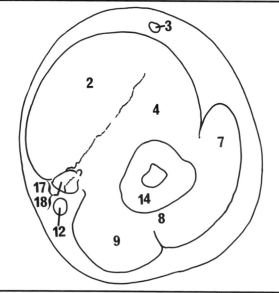

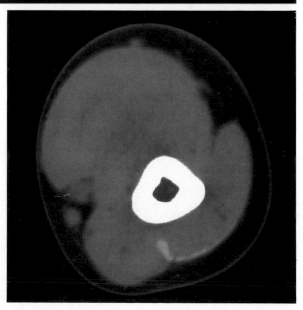

NOTES

This section passes through the mid-shaft of the humerus (14). It gives a clear view of the fascial arrangements of the upper arm; the investing sheath of the deep fascia (1) with its lateral (5) and medial (10) intermuscular septa which attach to the humeral shaft. These septa divide the extensor group of muscles, the triceps (7, 8, 9), from the anterior flexor group. The medial septum is pierced by the ulnar nerve (11) and its accompanying vessels (13), the lateral by the radial nerve with its accompanying profunda brachii artery and vein (6).

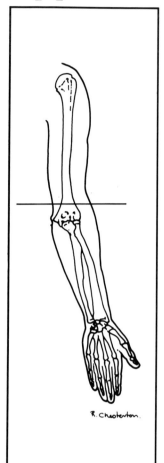

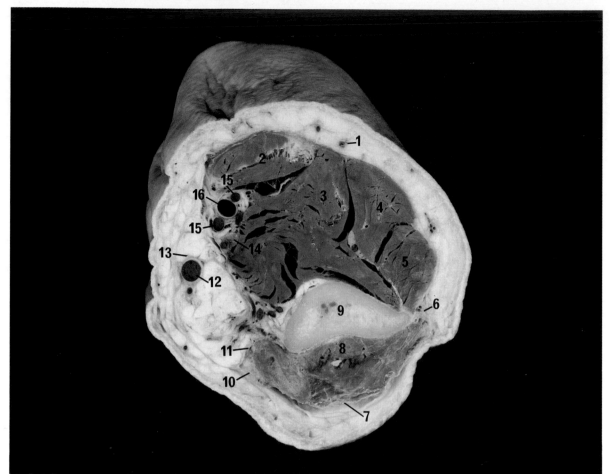

1 Cephalic vein
2 Biceps
3 Brachialis
4 Brachioradialis
5 Extensor carpi radialis longus
6 Lateral intermuscular septum
7 Triceps tendon
8 Triceps
9 Humerus
10 Ulnar nerve
11 Medial intermuscular septum
12 Basilic vein
13 Medial cutaneous nerve of forearm
14 Median nerve
15 Venae comitantes of brachial artery
16 Brachial artery

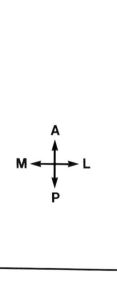

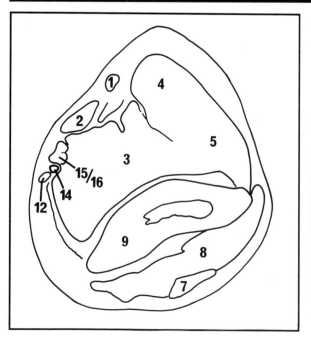

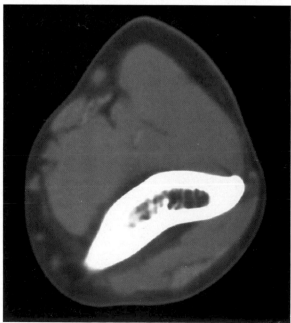

NOTES

This section transects the lower end of the humeral shaft as it expands to form its medial and lateral supracondylar ridges.

The origin of extensor carpi radialis longus (5) is from the upper part of the lateral ridge. This muscle arises superior to, and separate from, the remaining extensor muscles of the forearm, which come from a common origin from the lateral epicondyle of the humerus.

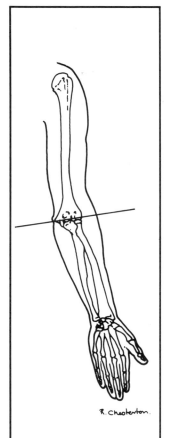

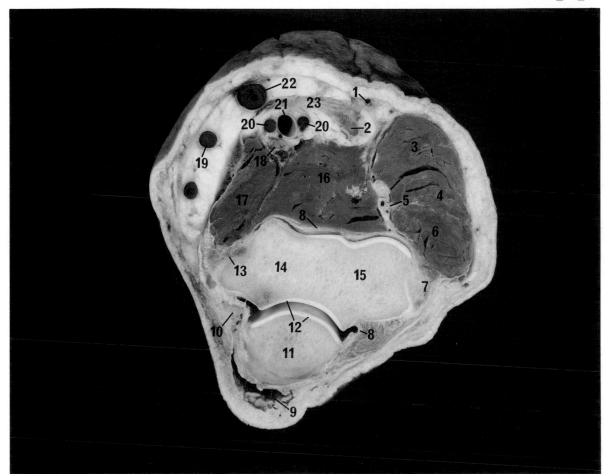

1 Cephalic vein
2 Biceps tendon
3 Brachioradialis
4 Extensor carpi radialis longus
5 Radial nerve with profunda brachii artery and vein
6 Common extensor origin
7 Lateral collateral ligament of elbow
8 Joint capsule of elbow
9 Olecranon bursa
10 Ulnar nerve
11 Olecranon process of ulna
12 Articular cartilage
13 Medial collateral ligament of elbow
14 Trochlea of humerus
15 Capitulum of humerus
16 Brachialis
17 Common flexor origin
18 Median nerve
19 Basilic vein
20 Venae comitantes of brachial artery
21 Brachial artery
22 Median cubital vein
23 Bicipital aponeurosis

24 Anconeus

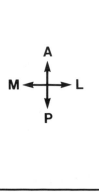

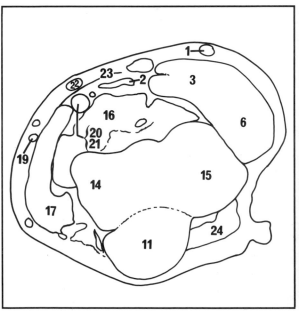

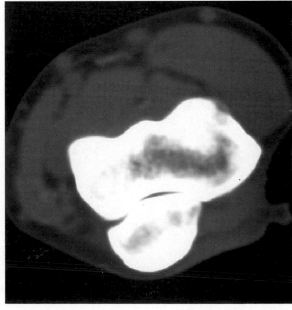

NOTES

This section transects the elbow joint.

The cartilage (12) covering the articular surfaces of the lower end of the humerus (14, 15) and the olecranon process of the ulna (11), together with the joint cavity and collateral ligaments (8) are readily appreciated.

The posterior surface of the olecranon process of the ulna is separated from the skin by a bursa (9). This is a common site for bursitis ('Student's elbow' or 'Miner's elbow').

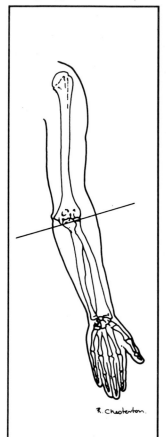

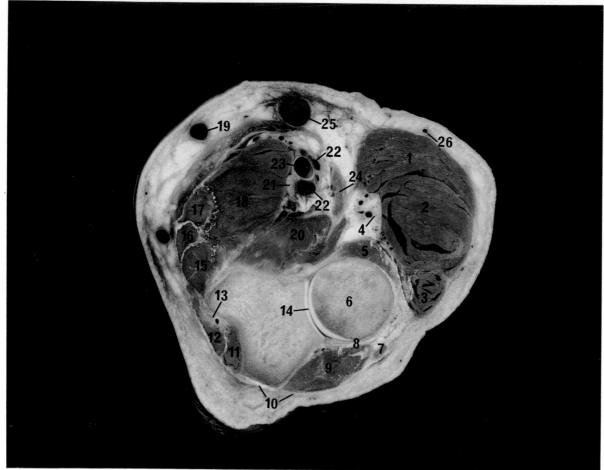

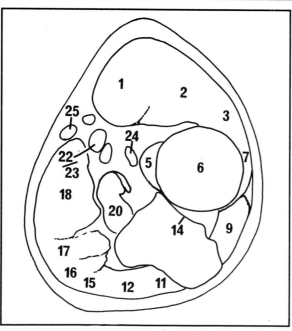

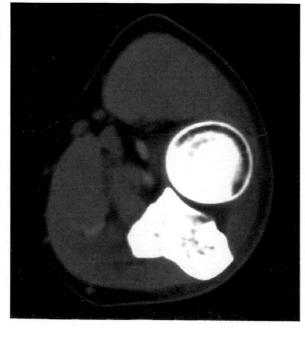

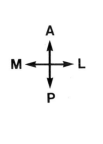

1 Brachioradialis
2 Extensor carpi radialis longus
3 Extensor carpi radialis brevis
4 Radial nerve with radial recurrent artery
5 Supinator
6 Head of radius
7 Common extensor origin
8 Annular ligament of superior radio-ulnar joint
9 Anconeus
10 Deep fascia of the forearm
11 Flexor digitorum profundus
12 Flexor carpi ulnaris
13 Ulnar nerve with posterior recurrent ulnar artery and vein
14 Radial notch of ulna
15 Flexor digitorum superficialis
16 Palmaris longus
17 Flexor carpi radialis
18 Pronator teres
19 Basilic vein
20 Brachialis
21 Median nerve
22 Venae comitantes of brachial artery
23 Brachial artery
24 Tendon of biceps
25 Median cubital vein
26 Cephalic vein

NOTES

This section passes through the superior radio-ulnar joint between the head of the radius (6) and the radial notch of the ulna (14). The annular ligament (8), which maintains the congruity of this pivot joint, is well shown. In the CT image the hand is in the neutral position alongside the body.

The median cubital vein (25) passes obliquely across the front of the elbow between the cephalic vein (26) and the basilic vein (19). It is separated from the underlying brachial artery (23) by a condensation of the deep fascia (10) termed the bicipital aponeurosis. Occasionally in high division of the brachial artery, an abnormal ulnar artery may lie immediately below the median cubital vein in the superficial fascia. This vein is therefore safer avoided for intravenous injections to protect against inadvertent intra-arterial injection.

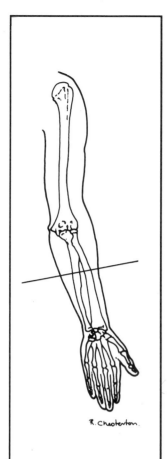

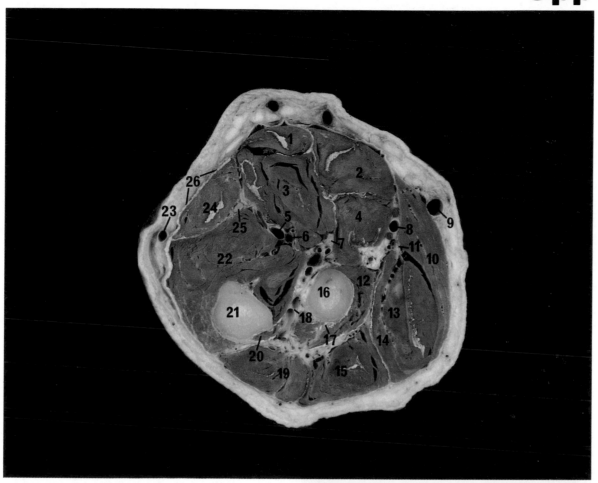

1 Palmaris longus
2 Flexor carpi radialis
3 Flexor digitorum superficialis
4 Pronator teres – humeral head
5 Ulnar artery
6 Ulnar vein
7 Median nerve with anterior interosseous artery and vein
8 Radial artery with venae comitantes
9 Cephalic vein
10 Brachioradialis
11 Radial nerve
12 Supinator
13 Extensor carpi radialis longus
14 Extensor carpi radialis brevis
15 Extensor digitorum
16 Radius
17 Posterior interosseous nerve
18 Posterior interosseous artery and vein
19 Extensor carpi ulnaris
20 Anconeus
21 Ulna
22 Flexor digitorum profundus
23 Basilic vein
24 Flexor carpi ulnaris
25 Ulnar nerve
26 Deep fascia of forearm

27 Pronator teres (ulnar head)

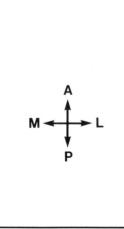

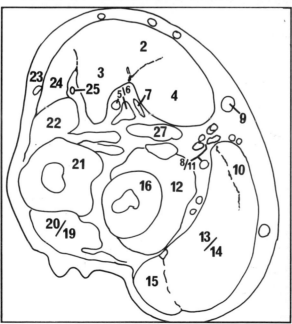

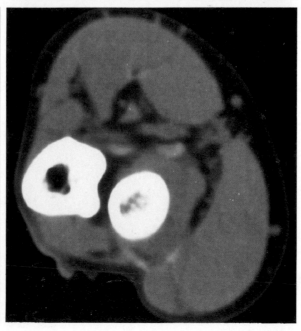

NOTES

This section passes through the mid forearm. In both the section and CT image the forearm is viewed in the supinated position.

Note how the median nerve (7) characteristically hugs the deep aspect of flexor digitorum superficialis (3). The ulnar nerve (25) lies sandwiched between flexor carpi ulnaris (24) and flexor digitorum profundus (22) and the radial nerve (11) lies beneath brachioradialis (10).

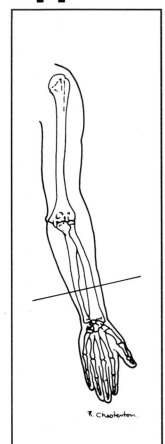

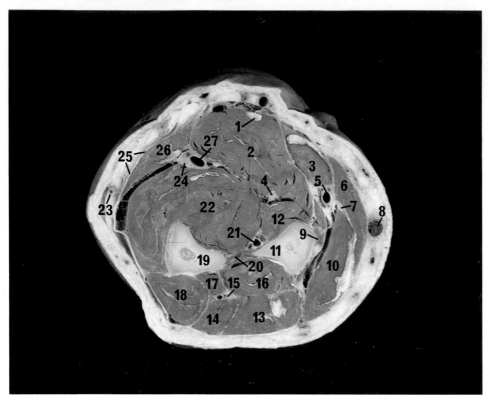

1 Palmaris longus tendon	16 Abductor pollicis longus
2 Flexor digitorum superficialis	17 Extensor pollicis longus
3 Flexor carpi radialis	18 Extensor carpi ulnaris
4 Median nerve	19 Ulna
5 Radial artery	20 Interosseous membrane
6 Brachioradialis	21 Anterior interosseous artery, vein and nerve
7 Radial nerve	22 Flexor digitorum profundus
8 Cephalic vein	23 Basilic vein
9 Pronator teres tendon	24 Ulnar nerve
10 Extensor carpi radialis longus and brevis	25 Deep fascia of forearm
11 Radius	26 Flexor carpi ulnaris
12 Flexor pollicis longus	27 Ulnar artery with venae comitantes
13 Extensor digitorum	
14 Extensor digiti minimi	28 Superficial flexor group of muscles
15 Posterior interosseous nerve with artery and vein	29 Extensor group of muscles

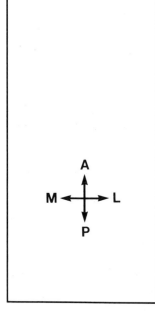

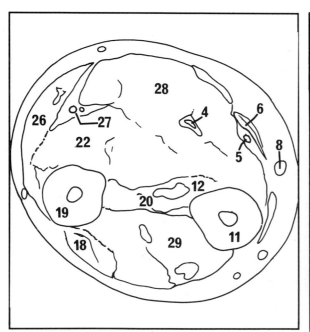

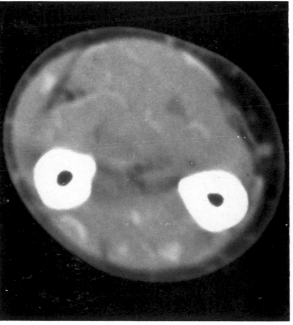

NOTES

This section transects the supinated forearm at the junction of its upper two-thirds and lower one-third.

Note that the very extensive origin of flexor digitorum profundus (22) is clearly demonstrated by this section. It arises from both the anterior and medial surfaces of the upper three quarters of the ulna (19), from the ulnar half of the interosseous membrane (20) and also from the superior three quarters of the posterior border of the ulna by an aponeurosis which is in common with that of flexor carpi ulnaris (26) and extensor carpi ulnaris (18).

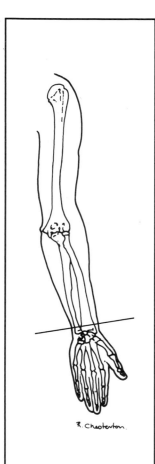

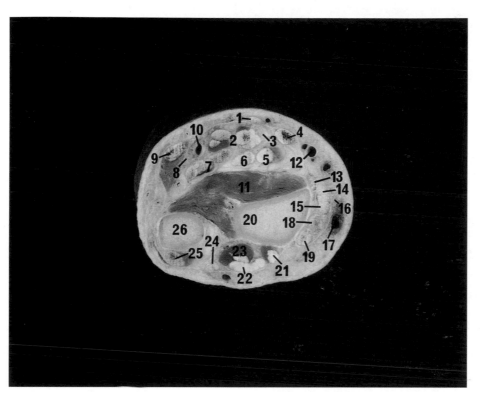

1 Palmaris longus tendon	15 Extensor pollicis brevis tendon
2 Flexor digitorum superficialis tendons	16 Radial nerve
3 Median nerve	17 Cephalic vein
4 Flexor carpi radialis tendon	18 Extensor carpi radialis longus tendon
5 Flexor pollicis longus tendon	19 Extensor carpi radialis brevis tendon
6 Flexor digitorum profundus tendon to index finger	20 Radius
7 Flexor digitorum profundus tendon to remaining fingers	21 Extensor pollicis longus tendon
	22 Extensor digitorum tendon
8 Ulnar nerve	23 Extensor indicis
9 Flexor carpi ulnaris tendon	24 Extensor digiti minimi tendon
10 Ulnar artery	25 Extensor carpi ulnaris tendon
11 Pronator quadratus	
12 Radial artery	26 Ulna
13 Brachioradialis insertion	
14 Abductor pollicis longus tendon	

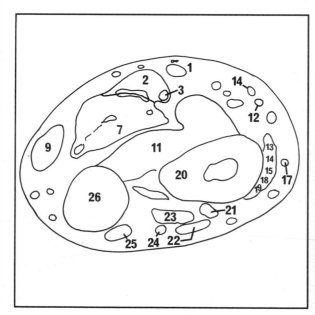

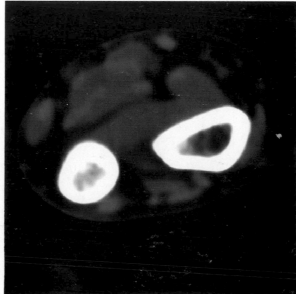

NOTES

This section transects the forearm immediately proximal to the wrist joint.

The arrangement of the extensor tendons on the posterior and radial aspects of the wrist can be clearly appreciated. Note that extensor carpi ulnaris tendon (25) grooves the dorsal aspect of the distal ulna (26).

At this level, flexor digitorum profundus has given off a separate tendon to the index finger (6) while those for the remaining three fingers are still closely applied to each other (7).

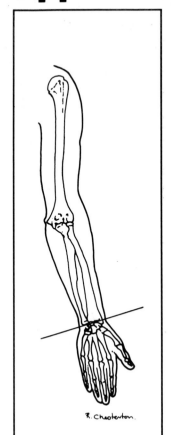

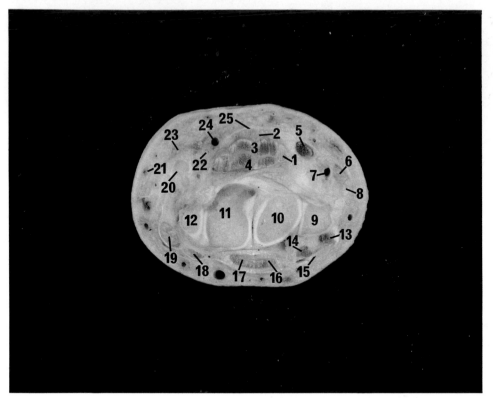

1 Flexor pollicis longus tendon	15 Extensor pollicis longus tendon
2 Median nerve	16 Extensor indicis tendon
3 Flexor digitorum superficialis tendons	17 Extensor digitorum tendon
4 Flexor digitorum profundus tendons	18 Extensor digiti minimi tendon
5 Flexor carpi radialis tendon	19 Extensor carpi ulnaris tendon
6 Abductor pollicis longus tendon	20 Pisiform
7 Radial artery	21 Basilic vein
8 Extensor pollicis brevis tendon	22 Ulnar nerve
9 Styloid process of radius	23 Flexor carpi ulnaris tendon
10 Scaphoid	24 Ulnar artery
11 Lunate	25 Flexor retinaculum
12 Triquetral	
13 Extensor carpi radialis longus tendon	26 Capitate
	27 Hamate
14 Extensor carpi radialis brevis tendon	28 Trapezoid
	29 Trapezium

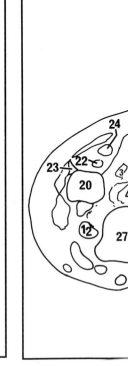

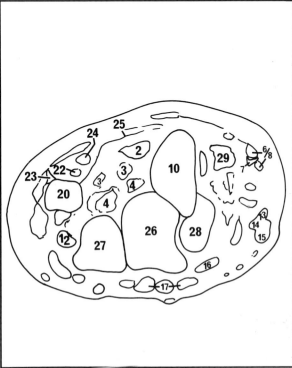

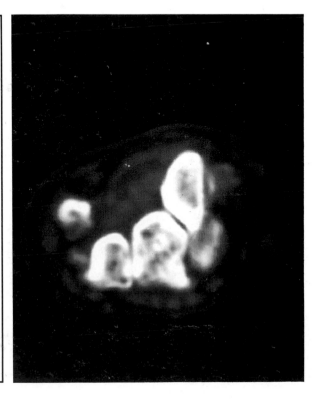

NOTES

This section passes through the proximal row of carpal bones and the radial styloid process. The CT image is at a more distal level.

The radius (9) extends more distally than the ulna; thus abduction of the wrist is more limited than adduction. The pisiform bone (20) can be considered as a sesamoid within the termination of the tendon of flexor carpi ulnaris (23), which anchors via the pisohamate ligament to the hook of the hamate and via the pisometacarpal ligament to the base of the fifth metacarpal bone.

The flexor retinaculum (25) is a tough fibrous band across the front of the carpus, which converts its concavity into the carpal tunnel, transmitting the flexor tendons of the digits together with the median nerve (2). Its attachments can be seen in this section and in section 88; medially to the pisiform (20) and to the hook of the hamate (27), laterally as two laminae, the more superficial one being attached to the tubercles of the scaphoid (10) and the trapezium (29) and the deep lamina to the medial lip of the groove on the latter.

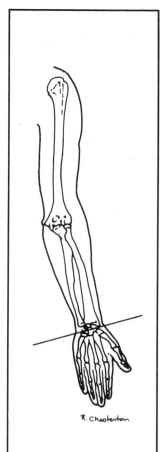

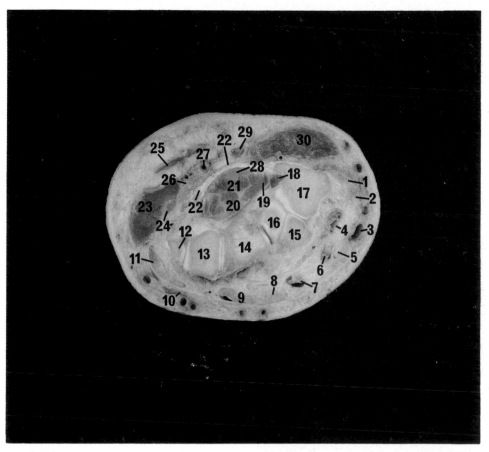

1 Abductor pollicis longus tendon	18 Flexor carpi radialis tendon
2 Extensor pollicis brevis tendon	19 Flexor pollicis longus tendon
3 Cephalic vein	20 Flexor digitorum profundus tendons
4 Radial artery	21 Flexor digitorum superficialis tendons
5 Extensor pollicis longus tendon	22 Flexor retinaculum
6 Extensor carpi radialis longus tendon	23 Muscles of hypothenar eminence
7 Extensor carpi radialis brevis tendon	24 Pisometacarpal ligament
8 Extensor indicis tendon	25 Palmaris brevis
9 Extensor digitorum tendon	26 Ulnar nerve
10 Extensor digiti minimi tendon	27 Ulnar artery
11 Extensor carpi ulnaris tendon	28 Median nerve
12 Triquetral	29 Palmaris longus tendon
13 Hamate	30 Muscles of thenar eminence
14 Capitate	
15 Trapezoid	31 First metacarpal base
16 Scaphoid	32 Second metacarpal base
17 Trapezium	33 Third metacarpal base
	34 Fourth metacarpal base
	35 Fifth metacarpal base

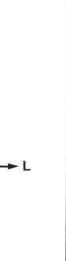

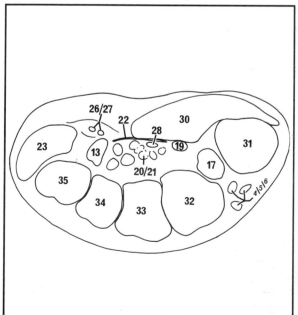

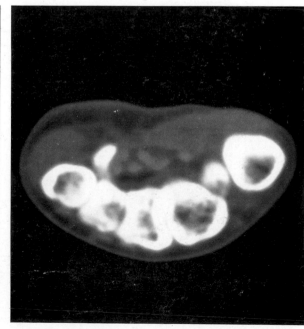

NOTES

This section passes through the distal part of the carpus and rather more distally, through the bases of the metacarpals on the CT image.

The flexor retinaculum (22) has already been described (see section 87). Here its distal attachment to the trapezium (17) and the hook of the hamate (13) can be seen. Note the tendon of flexor carpi radialis (18) lying in the tunnel formed by the groove on the trapezium and the two laminae of the lateral attachment of the retinaculum.

Swelling or deformity within the carpal tunnel compresses the median nerve (28) and produces the carpal tunnel syndrome.

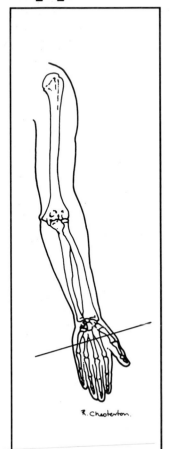

R. Chesterton.

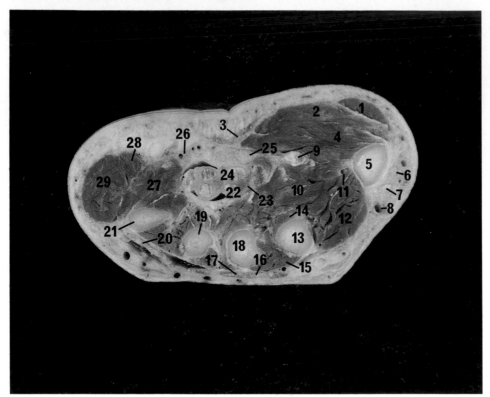

1 **Abductor pollicis brevis**	17 **Extensor digitorum tendon**
2 **Flexor pollicis brevis**	18 **Third metacarpal**
3 **Palmar aponeurosis**	19 **Fourth metacarpal**
4 **Oponens pollicis brevis**	20 **Extensor digiti minimi tendon**
5 **First metacarpal**	21 **Fifth metacarpal**
6 **Extensor pollicis brevis tendon**	22 **Flexor digitorum profundus tendons**
7 **Extensor pollicis longus tendon**	23 **Lumbrical**
8 **Cephalic vein**	24 **Flexor digitorum superficialis tendons**
9 **Flexor pollicis longus tendon**	25 **Median nerve**
10 **Adductor pollicis**	26 **Ulnar artery and nerve**
11 **Radial artery**	27 **Opponens digiti minimi**
12 **First dorsal interosseous**	28 **Flexor digiti minimi**
13 **Second metacarpal**	29 **Abductor digiti minimi**
14 **Second palmar interosseous**	
15 **Second dorsal interosseous**	30 **Muscles of thenar eminence**
16 **Extensor indicis tendon**	31 **Muscles of hypothenar eminence**

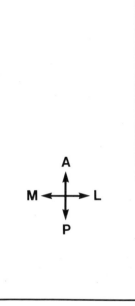

A
M ←→ L
P

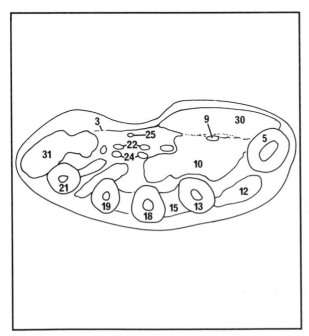

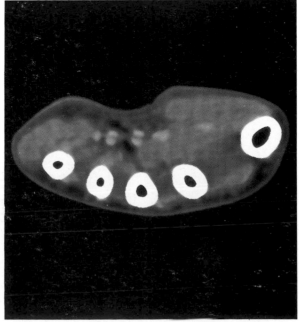

NOTES

This section passes through the proximal shafts of the metacarpals.

The dense central part of the palmar aponeurosis (3) is triangular, its apex being continuous with the distal margin of the flexor retinaculum (see sections 87 and 88). The expanded tendon of palmaris longus (see section 88) is attached to it. It is strongly bound to the overlying skin by dense fibroareolar tissue. Compare this with the loose superficial fascia over the extensor aspect of the hand. Oedema of the hand thus occurs only on its dorsal aspect. The lateral and medial extensions of the palmar aponeurosis are the thin superficial coverings of the thenar and hypothenar muscles respectively.

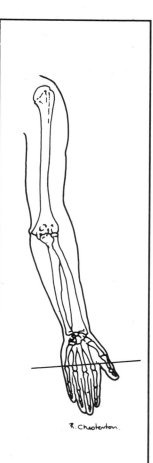

R. Chesterton.

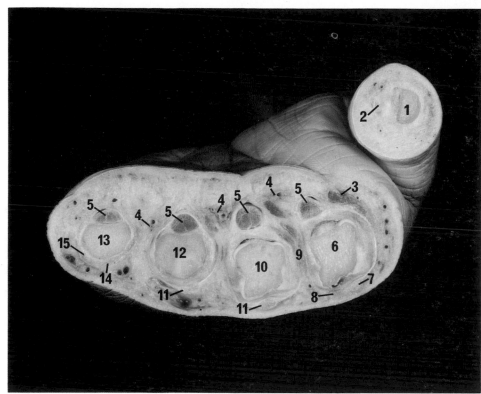

1 Proximal phalanx of thumb
2 Flexor pollicis longus tendon
3 First lumbrical
4 Neurovascular bundle
5 Flexor tendons within sheath
6 Second metacarpal head
7 Extensor digitorum tendon to index finger
8 Extensor indicis tendon
9 Interosseous muscles
10 Third metacarpal head
11 Extensor digitorum tendon
12 Fourth metacarpal head
13 Fifth metacarpal head
14 Extensor digitorum tendon to little finger
15 Extensor indicis tendon

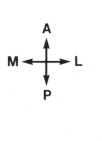

A
M ← → L
P

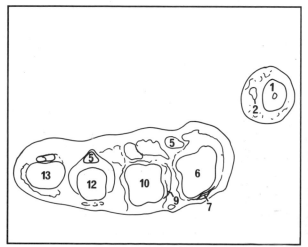

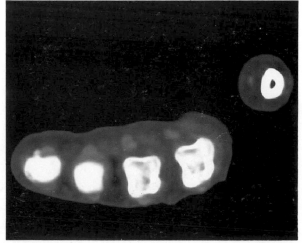

NOTES

This section passes through the heads of the metacarpals of the fingers and through the proximal phalanx of the thumb (1).

In the distal part of the palm, the digital arteries pass deeply between the divisions of the digital nerves so that, on the sides of the digits, the neurovascular bundle (4) has the digital nerve lying anterior to the digital artery and vein. The bundles lie adjacent to the tendon sheaths anterior to the metacarpal heads and this relationship is also maintained in the fingers. Thus an incision along the anterior border of the bone will avoid these important structures.

Index of notes